walk

WaLKING
SaN FraNCISCO

33 savvy tours exploring steep streets,
grand hotels, dive bars, and
waterfront parks

2nd Edition

Tom Downs

 WILDERNESS PRESS

Walking San Francisco: 33 savvy tours exploring steep streets, grand hotels, dive bars, and waterfront parks

2nd EDITION 2011
  3rd printing 2014

Copyright © 2011 by Tom Downs

Cover photos © 2011 by Tom Downs
Interior photos: Tom Downs, except for the following: Roslyn Bullas, pp. 203; Larry B. Van Dyke, 67 & 229
Maps: Bart Wright / Lohnes + Wright and Scott McGrew
Cover design: Larry B. Van Dyke and Scott McGrew
Book production: Annie Long
Book editor: Roslyn Bullas

ISBN 978-0-89997-654-9

Manufactured in the United States of America

Published by: **Wilderness Press**
                  Keen Communications
                  PO Box 43673
                  Birmingham, AL 35243
                  (800) 443-7227; FAX (205) 326-1012
                  info@wildernesspress.com
                  www.wildernesspress.com

Visit our website for a complete listing of our books and for ordering information.

Distributed by Publishers Group West

Cover photos: *Front, clockwise from bottom center:* Golden Gate Theater, Market Street; Diego Rivera's fresco, Russian Hill; Old U.S. Mint Building, South of Market; pagoda-style architecture, Chinatown; Washington Square Park, North Beach; Willie McCovey statue, China Park Basin; Golden Gate Bridge. *Back, clockwise from bottom left:* Chinatown Gate; Emporium rotunda, Market Street; Tadich Grill, Financial District.

Frontistpiece: Golden Gate Bridge from the Presidio

SAFETY NOTICE: Although Wilderness Press and the author have made every attempt to ensure that the information in this book is accurate at press time, they are not responsible for any loss, damage, injury, or inconvenience that may occur to anyone while using this book. You are responsible for your own safety and health while following the walking trips described here. Always check local conditions, know your own limitations, and consult a map.

acknowledgments

Many thanks to friends, family, and acquaintances who have informed and supported me along the way. My brother Jim, my sisters Kathy and Mary, my cousin Chris, and many of their friends, all introduced me to San Francisco when I was a teenager, which made me want to live in the city and get to know it. My wife Fawn and our kids Mai, Lana, and Liam regularly hit the pavement with me and rarely complain about taking the least direct route to wherever we're going. Mark Carrodus, John Fadeff, Beca Lafore, Randall Homan, Al Barna, and Rob Browne have all pulled my coat in one direction or another and have often accompanied me on walks. I owe a huge debt of gratitude to Roslyn Bullas and Heather Harrison at Wilderness Press, and to Holly Cross at Menasha Ridge.

author's note

All my life I have loved cities. As a kid, when watching cartoons or reading the so-called funny pages, I took an avid interest in the backdrops—the canyons of brick and mortar and the crevasses of glass and metal that were the stomping grounds of Superman, Batman, or Dick Tracy. That interest later merged into a love for film noir. Urban life—the great swarm of humanity, the incessant hush and groan machines, and constellations of electric light—grabbed hold of my imagination, and my curiosity has never been sated. I have lived contentedly in cities my entire adult life, and I spend a lot of time walking.

When I was young and scraping by, the streets were entertainment, and I took pride in knowing my environs. At first my walks were rambling, unwieldy explorations, which was exciting, but I found that the more I got to know about a city the more interesting I found the city to be. Walks, for me, became about place, about getting to know places.

Everything is relevant. Along with the feet, the mind must be permitted to ramble, to take everything in with equal interest. The walks in this book are grab bags of history, hard facts, anecdotes, and trivia all tied to the patch of geography known as San Francisco. Altogether, they are appreciations of a beautiful city.

While walking, use all the common sense you would usually have while strolling the streets of an American city. This book covers a lot of ground and is not limited to the hoitiest neighborhoods. That said, the only truly gritty district we'll walk through is the Tenderloin. Some parts of the Mission District also have their share of crime, but usually at night.

Perhaps the greatest caution should be exercised while doing the two bar-hopping tours in this book. On these walks, if you're not in your right mind, you're likely to stroll in front of a moving vehicle—or get shanghaied or something. Keep your wits about you, don't drink more than you can handle, and you'll be OK. Alright. Let's walk.

Numbers on this locator map correspond to Walk numbers.

TABLE OF CONTENTS

INTRODUCTION

San Francisco is a great walking city. It's a city of distinct neighborhoods, each with an intriguing history, beautiful buildings, and inviting places to eat or drink. That the city is far from flat may deter some, but rarely does San Francisco require a walker to trek up more than two steep blocks. Besides, reaching the top after an arduous climb comes with positive reinforcement, for the city's renowned beauty is fully realized only from the crests of its hills.

Most San Franciscans are accustomed to walking their city, but even city dwellers tend to have their familiar routes, which take them to where they need to go on a daily basis. This book invites locals and visitors to broaden their horizons, to explore well-trodden sidewalks at a slower pace, and to venture off onto the hidden corners of the city. These are not purposeful walks, but meandering, inquisitive strolls that focus on the story behind the buildings, the details that are easily missed if you're moving too fast, the unexpected detours down narrow alleys and behind unassuming doors where surprises await. The philosophy of this book is the pleasure is in getting there.

Broadway

Pacific Ave

Jackson St

Washington St

Clay St

Sacramento St

California St

Pine St

Bush St

Kearny St

Montgomery St

Sansome St

Battery St

Front St

Justin Herman Plaza

start

Ferry Building

Steuart St

Market St

Main St

Speal

EMBARCADERO

Powell St

Mason St

Sutter St

Post St

Stockton St

Grant Ave

MONTGOMERY ST

Fremont St

Beale St

1st St

Union Square

Geary St

O'Farrell St

POWELL ST

Yerba Buena Center for the Arts

2nd St

Ellis St

Eddy St

Turk Blvd

Leavenworth St

Jones St

Taylor St

Yerba Buena Gardens

Westfield San Francisco Centre

3rd St

Metreon

Moscone Center

4th St

Harrison St

80

Van Ness Ave

Polk St

Larkin St

Hyde St

CIVIC CENTER

Mission St

5th St

Howard St

6th St

Folsom St

Bryant St

Brannan St

finish

8th St

9th St

10th St

11th

7th St

80

King St

0   300   600   900 yards

0   300   600   900 meters

2

1 Lower Market Street: Wheeling, Dealing, and Hitting the Skids

BOUNDARIES: **Market St. from the Embarcadero to Van Ness Ave.**
DISTANCE: **2 miles**
DIFFICULTY: **Easy**
PARKING: **There's a parking garage at Embarcadero 2**
PUBLIC TRANSIT: **Embarcadero BART station; F streetcars (street level); J, K, L, M, N, S streetcars (underground); 1, 2, 14, 21, 71 Muni buses**

Market St. slices through San Francisco's grid at a brash, oblique angle, cutting a prominent seam through the city's central neighborhoods. It is a direct conduit into the city from San Francisco's historic entrepot, the Ferry Building, leading all the way to Twin Peaks, where it heads skyward and disappears, having vaguely shown the way to the Pacific Ocean without actually leading there. It serves as the city's parade ground, but Market doesn't require a parade to be interesting. To walk this graceful corridor on a weekday morning is to be urged along by the living thrum of an American city. Muni buses, taxis, restored streetcars, autos, and bicycles generate a deep-throated hush as their wheels roll up and down Market's lanes. The street's swift-footed office workers swerve to avoid statues, fountains, and historical markers, as well as the casual sightseer who stops to inspect these monuments of the street's stately past. Billions in U.S. dollars have been earned, lost, and swindled in the high-rise and flatiron structures along blocks that hem the Financial District, and billions more have been spent in the emporiums near Union Square. West of the Powell St. cable car turnaround, Market St. once thrived as San Francisco's Broadway, with two or three grand theaters to a block. Some survive today, but this stretch of the city's main thoroughfare, up to Van Ness, has seen much better days. The contrast from one end of this walk to the other is striking and, in some ways, baffling. All in all, a walk along Market St. makes a fine introduction to San Francisco. This walk is as straightforward as they come.

● **Start at the foot of Market St., opposite the Ferry Building and separated from the Embarcadero by just a few paces. (The Ferry Building is explored in greater detail in the Embarcadero North walk.) The open space here is Justin Herman Plaza, named for the controversial head of San Francisco's Redevelopment Agency from 1959** to 1971. (Herman is generally held accountable for the displacement of thousands of black residents in the Western Addition as that neighborhood was subjected to extensive renewal projects during the early 1960s.) For decades, this awkward plaza was marred by the elevated Embarcadero Freeway, which ran along the bayfront, until the 1989 Loma Prieta earthquake brought it down. Today the plaza is a pleasant space, with palm trees, an open-air crafts market, and live music several days a week around lunchtime. At the plaza's northeastern corner is homely Villaincourt Fountain, described by the late *San Francisco Chronicle* architecture critic Allan Temko as something "deposited by a concrete dog with square intestines." Nevertheless, steps through the fountain's shallow pool invite you to venture behind the huge spouts, where you're likely to get a wee bit wet while enjoying a backstage perspective. This is a good vantage of the staggered backside of the Hyatt Regency hotel. (The Embarcadero Center, which also towers over the plaza, is included in the Financial District walk.)

● Start walking up Market St., noting the attractive One Market building across the street. It was home base for the Southern Pacific Railroad, the enormous conglomerate run by the Big Four railroad magnates, who dominated transportation in the Western U.S. during the late 19th century. The building went up in 1916. SP survived until 1996, when the company was absorbed by Union Pacific.

● At Drumm St., turn right and enter the Hyatt Regency, which is merely interesting from the outside but looks truly spectacular from within. Head up the escalator to the Atrium level, where glass elevators whiz up to tiered, vertigo-inducing balconies. Mel Brooks took full advantage of the striking setting when he shot scenes for *High Anxiety* here. Ride an elevator up and down and get back to Market St.

● Cross over to the other side at Spear. The high arcade arching halfway over the sidewalk here is part of the Federal Reserve Bank, completed in 1983. Inside, the Fed Center exhibits explore the theme of money and banking, with a currency collection dating back to colonial days.

● The next block is dominated by the Matson and PG&E buildings, which make a perfect pair. The Matson office, home to the city's largest shipping line, was built in 1921, and the office of the local power company, PG&E, went up four years later. Scan the ledges of the upper floors of these buildings and you might spot one of the peregrine falcons that regularly perch there. From 2003–05, two falcons, dubbed Gracie and George, raised their nestlings outside the 33rd floor of the PG&E Building, overlooking Beale St. More recently another pair, Dapper Dan and Diamond Lil, have nested on the same ledge. Peregrines are often seen amid the high rises of Market St.

● If you look back across Market St., you'll get an eyeful of 101 California St., a cylindrical glass tower that's worth a closer look. Cross over to it, and you'll see that the lower floors are supported by unclad pillars. The exposed pillars, which of course run unseen to the top of the building, look naked and suspiciously vulnerable without the glass curtain. Unfortunately, 101 California is known mostly as the scene of a senseless murder-suicide. On July 1, 1993, John Luigi Ferri, a disgruntled claimant, entered the law offices of Pettit & Martin, on the 34th floor, and gunned down eight employees before killing himself. Six others were wounded in the attack.

At the confluence of Market, Battery, and Bush streets, breaking office workers and bike messengers often perch at the base of the *Mechanics Monument* statue, a robust bronze by Douglas Tilden, who was educated at San Francisco's Deaf and Dumb and Blind Asylum. (He was deaf.) The statue was unveiled in 1901 to some protest from those who observed that the subjects—muscular ironworkers—were not wearing pants beneath their blacksmith aprons, leaving their bums exposed to the elements. Tilden, himself regarded as the Michelangelo of the West, argued he was observing the classical ideal. The nude ironworkers may have had their hams roasted during the 1906 quake and fire, but were otherwise little harmed.

● Midway across Battery, on the little triangular island, keep your eyes peeled for a historical marker that informs us that the slot machine was invented by Charles August Fey in his workshop near this spot in 1894. For the better part of a century, Fey's three-reel, hand-cranked "one-armed bandit" was the slot machine of choice in many a Nevada casino. The green-tinted glass curtain wall that towers over the next block (between Battery and Sansome) is the Crown-Zellerbach Building. Built in 1959, it's one of San Francisco's most attractive modern buildings.

Market St.'s triangular corners necessitated the design of numerous flatiron buildings, so called because they are shaped like the old blockish irons long ago heated on stoves before being applied to wrinkled shirts. Modern office towers such as the Crown-Zellerbach Building often flout the shape of their lots with surrounding plazas and whatnot, but the next block is occupied by a traditional flatiron building of the sort that once lined much of Market St. This tasteful flatiron dates to 1913.

● On the same block, toward the wider end, stands the Hobart Building, an attractive 1914 Willis Polk design. Part of the building's unintended appeal comes from the fact that its design took a shorter adjacent neighbor into account. When that building was demolished and replaced by an even shorter structure, the Hobart Building's flat western flank was awkwardly exposed. In any case, it's still lovely to look at.

● Cross Market St. and glance back for a better perspective of the Hobart Building before heading half a block up New Montgomery to the main entrance of the Palace Hotel. It was built in 1909 on the site of the far more magnificent original Palace, which was destroyed by the '06 fire. The Palace is still spectacular, especially the atrium with its Victorian glass roof. Go inside for a look, or for an expensive pot of tea in the atrium, and exit via a hall leading back to Market St. On your way out, you'll pass the Pied Piper bar. If it's open, peek inside for a look at the mural by Maxfield Parrish. If you're a mite parched you can stop for a beer as well.

● Another block up, at the corner of 3rd and Market, is the Hearst Building, its entry marked by a big "H." Built in 1909, it was home to William Randolf Hearst's *San Francisco Examiner*. Julia Morgan designed the building's Baroque entry, which was added in 1937. During the early 20th century, this intersection was home to two of the city's other leading papers, the *Call* and the *Chronicle*. The Call Building has been remodeled beyond recognition, its once glorious dome having been removed to accommodate additional floors. But the *Chronicle*'s old home, the de Young Building (1890) at 690 Market, has been restored and resembles its former self. Designed by Burnham and Root, it originally sported a four-story clock tower, which went up in smoke a year before the 1906 quake. In the 1960s the entire building was covered with metal siding, which obscured the building's solid brick appeal. As part of its recent restoration, a modern tower was added awkwardly to the top of this graceful landmark, but is set back enough not to detract from the attractive façade.

In front of the de Young Building you'll spot Lotta's Fountain, legendary for the congregations that gather here every year on April 18 to commemorate the 1906 earthquake. The festivities traditionally include a few quake survivors, whose numbers are obviously dwindling. In 2009 a 106-year-old woman and a 103-year-old man were

Back Story: Palatial Intrigue

The original Palace Hotel was the center of the city's social life and the downfall of William Ralston, the banker who literally went belly up while building it. First Ralston went bankrupt and then he died while swimming in the bay, a few weeks before the hotel's opening. Many suspect it was a suicide.

Three decades later, opera star Enrico Caruso, in town to perform in a production of *Carmen*, stayed in the old Palace the night of April 17, 1906. Just after 5 a.m. the following morning, Caruso evacuated the shaking building several hours before flames engulfed it. Some eye-witnesses claimed the singer was in an embarrassing state of panic, but Caruso wrote a lengthy account for a London publication refuting this attack on his character. He admitted he and his valet wandered helplessly about the city, as did thousands of others, as the entire downtown area went up in smoke. He slept on the ground on the night of April 18 and found his way out of town the following day. He never returned to San Francisco.

On August 2, 1923, President Warren G. Harding—remembered for the corruption in his cabinet and for his poor command of the English language—died at the rebuilt Palace Hotel after he was stricken with what was thought to be food poisoning while traveling to the city from Alaska. Mysteriously, no one Harding had dined with got sick, and conspiracy theories abounded. The official cause of death was later deemed a heart attack.

in attendance. In the aftermath of the quake, the fountain was a meeting place for separated families. It was a gift to the city in 1875 from Lotta Crabtree (1847–1924), a beguiling redhead who as a child entertainer worked the halls of Sierra Nevada mining towns. When she matured she moved East and became the "Belle of Broadway."

● At the intersection of Market, Grant, and O'Farrell streets is the Phelan Building, a large and elegant flatiron. Clad in white terra-cotta tiles, it's one of the prettiest sights on all of Market St. James Duvall Phelan, the city's mayor from 1897 to 1902 and a U.S. Senator from 1915 to 1921, kept his offices here after the building went up in 1908.

● Cross Market St. and walk on the south side. Midway up the next block, enter Westfield Centre, a shopping mall fashioned from the gutted shell of the historic Emporium department store. The façade is original, as is the beautiful glass rotunda, which is the building's real attraction. You'll have to work to see it, though, as it is obscured by intermediary levels and escalators.

● Across the street, the block is dominated by the grey hulk of the Flood Building, built by James L. Flood, son of the Silver King James C. Flood. It's an impressive eye-catcher with a staunch demeanor. In the early 1920s, Dashiell Hammett, yet to establish himself as the father of American crime fiction, worked upstairs for the local branch of the Pinkerton Detective Agency. Today, as you'll see, its ground floor houses a Gap flagship store.

● Just past Halladie Plaza and the Powell St. cable car turnaround (launching point of the Union Square Walk), Market St. begins to change noticeably. Here, many storefronts are covered with plywood and POST NO BILLS signs. Shops still operating on the next block include a discount luggage store, a Western Union, and the Crazy Horse Gentlemen's Club, its sign featuring the sort of reclining long-haired women usually found on the mud flaps of 18-wheelers. The Warfield, between Mason and Taylor, and the Golden Gate Theatre, where Taylor and Golden Gate meet Market, are still important venues for live music and Broadway shows.

● Past 6th St., the building at 1017–21 Market, with immense fluted pillars and oversized windows in front, is very stately and, on the ground level, empty. It was designed in 1909 by George Applegarth, who had a fondness for glass fronts long before they became the norm. A few doors down, the Market Street Cinema has seen better days, going all the way back to 1912 when it opened as Grauman's Imperial. Its gaudy marquee is ever changing, but on a recent fall morning it made the following pitch: FOOTBALL SEASON IS GETTING STARTED! WHY NOT COME IN AND FACE OUR FRONT LINE OF FULLY NUDE SHOW GIRLS AND BE SURE TO GO THE EXXXTRA YARD TO MAKE THAT TOUCHDOWN.

● Kaplan's Gov't Surplus has its smartly abbreviated name spelled out in chipped letters on a decrepit sign. It has been in business since 1939. The store's windows display a broadly diverse array of merchandise, including a selection of sneakers and military footwear, $3 sunglasses, Kangol caps, authentic-looking San Francisco

Giants' jerseys with pitcher Tim Lincecum's name and number on the back, Dickie stretch pants, cheap plastic cigarette lighters, a box of ancient-looking sewing awls, a box of genuine leather tri-fold wallets priced at $4.99 apiece, a Ben Davis sign with the brand's smiling monkey logo, bullet key chains, camo handkerchiefs, camo belts with ratchet buckles, a selection of quilted camo vests in brown and green and grey, polyester U.S. flags, and T-shirts with SECURITY printed on the front. There's a sure-fire formula for longevity on a topsy turvy street.

- The Hibernia Bank Building, designed by Albert Pissis and William Moore in 1892, dominates the intersection of Jones, McAllister, and Market. The building hasn't housed a bank since the mid 1980s. Over the next decade, it was home to the SFPD's Tenderloin Task Force, which departed in 2000. It is a lovely building, with a green copper dome, and after long neglect it is finally being fixed up, though to what purpose is not yet clear. Talk of turning the building into a museum or a juvenile court quieted down a few years ago.

- On the next block, with a little loving care, the Renoir Hotel, a flatiron clad in brick, looks promising. The hip-looking lounge on the ground floor has a hand-painted sign out front that says LOVE WILL SOLVE ALL YOUR PROBLEMS and below that, written upside down, LOVE WILL ONLY LET YOU DOWN.

- At 7th St. the sturdy Grant Building, a steel-framed quake survivor, and the comely Odd Fellows Temple, where Odd Fellows still congregate, face off on opposite corners. Also at this intersection are steps leading down to the below-ground Civic Center BART station, a check-cashing outlet, an uninviting eatery called the Oriental Restaurant, and a striking view of City Hall via U.N. Plaza's diagonal open space. Next to the Dollar Market, the National Hotel has an unadorned brick façade that has been quake proofed with prominent metal braces. A sign advertises unspecified NITELY & WEEKLY RATES. Judging by the hotel's front windows, which are filled with plants, candles, and cans of food, the place is well settled into.

- A few doors down, on the ground floor of One Trinity Center, Caffè Trinity is a beautiful little spot that's easily missed. Enter the marble and wood interior for a warm drink and take advantage of the cafe's cozy cove seating.

● Past U.N. Plaza, the Orpheum Theater has a spruced up, flamboyant façade that's at odds with the downtrodden state of affairs around it. Built in 1926, the Orpheum was initially a Pantages vaudeville theater and then a grand movie palace. Today, it houses Broadway stage productions. Step into the covered entryway, elegantly clad in marble. It's still a beauty.

● On the other side of Market, the Trinity Plaza Apartments look almost empty, and may have been demolished by the time you walk this block. A sign in front says NOW RENTING—but this surely refers to the new tower around the block. For years, the building's owners have tried to demolish it and replace it with a complex of much larger towers that will likely include 1,700 apartments and street-level retail space. The plan is to move this building's tenants into rent-controlled apartments in the new tower, then complete the redevelopment plan on this Market St. location. In the balance is the direction this part of Market St. will likely take in the years ahead.

● Past 8th St., a plaque beside the entrance of the Hotel Whitecomb states that the hotel served as City Hall from 1912–15, while the current City Hall was being built. The rest of the block is occupied by a cold office tower that from the street appears devoid of life. Few walk in or out even during the busiest of times. Kitty corner to that, at 9th St., Fox Plaza, a mix of offices and rental apartments, is similarly off-putting. Unwelcoming high-rises such as these reflect a regrettable mid-century approach to redevelopment, which all too often failed to bring renewed energy to the surrounding neighborhood. In this case, as a twist to the knife, Fox Plaza stands on the site of the long lamented Fox Theatre, a stunning movie palace that was demolished in 1963. Across from Fox Plaza, the block-long SF Mart Building has an appealing early-20th-century style, though its face is somewhat monotonous. It doesn't help that the building's shop fronts are sealed off with painted plywood, further contributing to the lifeless feel of this stretch of Market.

● The intersection of Market and 10th streets has a vacant lot, a youth hostel, and a sleek new high-rise apartment building, 1 Polk, that may be an indication of future things to come. However, banners on the front of this new tower—NOW LEASING, MOVE IN TODAY—seem a bit eager. It may be a while before the well-heeled clamor to move into this neighborhood.

- On the next block, a drab building at 1444 Market is surrounded with police barricades, long after a hundred law enforcement agents raided the place in August 1996. It is the former home of the Cannabis Buyers' Club, which had begun operating before medical marijuana had been legalized in the state of California.

- A few doors down is the corner of Van Ness Ave., and the end of this walk.

POINTS OF INTEREST

Hyatt Regency 5 Embarcadero Center, 415-788-1234

Federal Reserve Bank (Fed Center) 101 Market St., 415-974-3252

Palace Hotel (Pied Piper Bar) 2 New Montgomery St., 415-512-1111

Caffè Trinity 1145 Market St., 415-626-2346

ROUTE SUMMARY

1. Begin at the foot of Market St., opposite the Ferry Building.
2. Head up one block to Drumm St. and hook right into the Hyatt Regency.
3. Continue up Market St. to New Montgomery, turn left, walk half a block to enter Palace Hotel.
4. Inside the Palace Hotel, walk to Garden Court, then follow hall back to Market St.
5. Continue on Market to Van Ness Ave.

Hyatt Regency

Lombard St

Pioneer Park

The Embarcadero

Filbert St

Alta St

Union St

Union St

Sansome St

Battery St

Green St

San Francisco Bay

Vallejo St

Pier 7

Montgomery St

Broadway St

Front St

Davis St

Walton Square

Pacific Ave

Jackson St

The Embarcadero

Columbus Ave

Washington St

Embarcadero Plaza

Ferry Building

Merchant St

finish

Maritime Plaza

start

Clay St

Davis St

Drumm St

Justin Herman Plaza

| 0 | 100 | 200 | 300 yards |
| 0 | 100 | 200 | 300 meters |

Sacramento St

2 eMBarcadero NortH: coverING THe waterfront

BOUNDARIES: **Market St., Embarcadero, Chestnut St., Sansome St.**
DISTANCE: **2¼ miles**
DIFFICULTY: **Easy**
PARKING: **There is off-street parking at the Embarcadero Center and on Howard St.**
PUBLIC TRANSIT: **Embarcadero BART station; F streetcar; J, K, L, M, and N Muni underground trains; 14 Muni bus**

Much of the history of early San Francisco centered on the waterfront around Yerba Buena Cove, which before it was filled in curved into what is now the Financial District, as far inland as Battery St. At high tide, early structures along Montgomery St. are said to have had water lapping at their steps. Most of the ground we'll tread on this tour covers the bones of rotted ships, many of which were abandoned by seamen who made a dash for the diggings in the Sierra foothills. Some deserted ships became boarding houses, while others were converted into saloons. One even served as the city jail. Eventually, their wooden hulls formed the foundation for landfill, and the wharves where they tied on became the city streets we walk today.

For the unwary sailor, a stop in this neighborhood was perilous indeed, with swindlers and crimps seeming friendly enough until the hapless seaman was drugged or slugged and sold to the next ship embarking on a two-year voyage. This practice was prevalent in other ports, but it ran rampant in San Francisco, where it became known as "shanghaiing." We'll uncover some of that history here, so keep your wits about ye.

This tour doesn't dwell exclusively on the past, though, for the Embarcadero is returning to life after its late 20th century slumber. Saturday morning, when the Ferry Building Farmers' Market is on, is a good time to begin this tour.

● **Begin at the Ferry Building. Built in 1898, the Ferry Building instantly established itself as the principal entryway to the city, and it remained so until bridges and airplanes made it possible to arrive in San Francisco from the east without taking a ride on a ferry boat. For a time it was one of the busiest transit hubs in the world, with some 100,000 passengers passing through every day. Ferry traffic began to diminish after the completion of the Bay Bridge in 1936. The building's dwindling importance**

Back Story: Shanghaiing

Among San Francisco's gifts to the English language is "shanghai," the verb. Sailors put aboard ships against their will were said to have been "shanghaied" by crimps who made a good living through such dastardly deeds. Bill Pickelhaupt, in his book *Shanghaied in San Francisco*, nicely explains the term's etymology. According to Pickelhaupt, during the mid-19th century, Shanghai, China, was not on direct shipping routes from San Francisco, so a sea voyage to that port necessarily involved an indirect course around the globe lasting about two years before a sailor returned to San Francisco. Sailors almost always had to be persuaded, honestly or otherwise, to accept such assignments.

In San Francisco, a perpetual shortage of seamen—often due to the opportunities and distractions available in the boisterous boom town and at the gold fields—led to an increase in crimping. Crimps sold unconscious sailors to shipping companies in return for the sailors' first two months of wages. Most often the destination was not actually Shanghai. Though the practice was illegal, politicians and businessmen saw the value in looking the other way, and crimps with names like Shanghai Kelly and Shanghai Chicken Devine felt no need to hide the nature of their business. Kelly's knockout cocktail, served in his saloon, was a mixture of schnapps, beer, and a narcotic—usually opium.

was obvious by the time the elevated Embarcadero Freeway was completed in 1959, effectively concealing much of the Ferry Building from the rest of the city. That proved to be a temporary problem, solved by the 1989 earthquake, which damaged the elevated freeway. The freeway was demolished a few years later, giving new life to the Ferry Building. Thus, the landmark has survived the 1906 earthquake, the demise of ferry traffic, the intrusion of a freeway, and the 1989 quake. Its has been restored, and the ground floor has been repurposed as an atmospheric marketplace with shops and eateries specializing in gourmet foods. The Ferry Building Marketplace takes the shopping mall food court concept to a new level, with a tasteful style that appeals to locals and tourists alike. When the farmers' market is on (Tuesday and Thursday 10 a.m.–2 p.m., Saturday 8 a.m.–2 p.m.) the Ferry Plaza and Marketplace bustle with vendors and crowds of people indulging in San Francisco's passionate culture of food.

Walk through the building and around it, past the benches offering front-row views of the bay, Treasure Island, the Bay Bridge, and the Port of Oakland beyond. The fine Slanted Door, a modern Vietnamese restaurant, anchors the dining scene here. Ferries continue to launch here, too.

● Exit the front of the Ferry Building and turn right onto the Embarcadero, which has also been dubbed Herb Caen Way to commemorate the legendary columnist for the *San Francisco Chronicle* and *Examiner*. Caen was fond of calling the city "Baghdad by the Bay," and he famously resuscitated Emperor Norton's 19th-century ban on calling the city "Frisco." The Baghdad tag has proved a bad fit, but many San Franciscans remain quick to censure anyone for the use of "Frisco." Caen wrote his anecdotal column, rife with insider knowledge and ellipses, for some 60 years until his death in February 1997.

● Just past Pier 3, near the foot of Broadway, is the Pier 7 pedestrian wharf, which extends 900 feet out into the bay. Walk out and you're likely to encounter anglers extending fishing poles over the sides. You may even see someone net a rock crab, which they are entitled to take home for dinner, or a Dungeness crab, which by law they are required to throw back. The pier, built in 1990, juts out into the bay in roughly the spot where ships docked at the old Broadway Pier. Piers extended out from Vallejo and Pacific streets as well. Running perpendicular to these piers, Front St. stood on wooden pilings driven into the mud of the bay as late as the mid-1860s. Boardinghouses and saloons crowded around the wharves in a town still short on housing and women. You'll need to use your imagination to picture any of this today, but a few buildings from that period survive along the course of this walk.

● At Pier 15, you're likely to spot a few tractor tugs operated by Baydelta Maritime. On the sidewalk here, look for a historical marker entitled BARBARY COAST, which has some tasty excerpts from author Herbert Asbury and historian H. H. Bancroft, describing the rough-and-tumble entertainment district that was centered along Pacific Ave. just west of here.

A little ways down the Embarcadero, the Pier 23 Cafe is a basic, squat wooden shack on the wharf, with seafood, a bar, and live music most nights. Sunday afternoon, when live jazz is performed from 4 p.m. to 8 p.m., is a popular time to drop by, especially when the weather is agreeable and you can relax on the back patio overlooking the bay. Just beyond the restaurant, Pier 23 itself still functions as a warehouse for goods shipped in from overseas. If the gates are open, you'll spot pallets loaded up with imported goods, mostly from the People's Republic of China.

● Cross the Embarcadero at Lombard or Chestnut St. and have a look at the Fog City Diner, a spangly reinterpretation of the traditional East Coast diner. The food here is also a reinterpretation, with the kitchen applying some of the principles of California Cuisine to classic fare served up in diners and seafood grills.

● From the diner, follow Battery St. a few paces and detour into the small public space behind it, following the path through the little stream and fountain. This is an extension of Levi Strauss Plaza, corporate headquarters for the company that put blue jeans on the legs of the world. German-born Levi Strauss came to San Francisco in 1853 and opened a dry goods shop. In 1870, he and Jacob Davis, a tailor, patented durable canvas work pants on which the seams were reinforced with copper rivets, a distinguishing trademark. Cut through the center of the campus-like office complex, built in the early 1980s. It incorporates modern structures along with a pair of stately warehouses dating to the early 1900s. At Sansome St. turn left.

● Two blocks down, in the nondescript industrial structure at 200 Green St., Philo T. Farnsworth invented television. Farnsworth, a native of Utah, publicly demonstrated his invention for the first time in 1927. He lived until 1971, long enough to have watched broadcasts of *Mr. Ed, The Mod Squad,* and the landing of Apollo 11 on the moon.

    The corner of Sansome and Green was the northeastern extent of a neighborhood known during the Gold Rush as Sydney Town (sometimes spelled with a hyphen), largely inhabited by ticket-of-leave men from Australia. The denizens of this menacing little fun-zone, which extended west to Kearny and south to Broadway, were known as the Sydney Ducks, and by and large were considered to be ruffians or worse by the rest of San Francisco. On several occasions large portions of the city burned to the ground and Australians were blamed for kindling the flames or for plundering in the wake of disaster. Many were executed by vigilantes. The Committee of Vigilance of 1851 was formed in large part to contain the outlaw activities of Sydney Town residents.

● At Vallejo St. turn left and continue to Front St. The building on the corner, at 855 Front St., is the Daniel Gibb warehouse, built in 1855. It's a rare Gold Rush era survivor built on landfill at the shore of the bay. Gibb was an importer of goods ranging from liquor to coal. It now is an office building, but looks much as it would have 150 years ago.

- Follow Front St. down to Pacific Ave. and turn right. At Battery, the Old Ship Saloon is a lovely old bar with a dark past. This establishment has an indelible link to James Laflin, one of the city's most notorious shanghaiers. The building dates to 1907 but stands where the business has stood since 1851. The establishment was originally in an old ship, the *Arkansas,* which was abandoned by a crew excited by news of gold strikes. The *Arkansas* docked here and her forecastle was transformed into a drinking tavern before Yerba Buena Cove was filled. Laflin sailed over on the *Arkansas* as a cabin boy and became a bartender in the Old Ship Saloon. He soon gained infamy as one of the city's most successful crimps, selling unconscious seamen to ships sailing out in the morning. A model of a ship, standing in for the *Arkansas,* hangs over the street corner, above the bar's main entrance. Have a drink here—you probably won't end up in Shanghai.

- Turn left onto Battery, then left again at Jackson. Enter the old portals to Sydney Walton Square, now an open space but once the sight of numerous saloons. The Boston House, run by James "Shanghai" Kelly, whose notoriety circled the globe, stood at 33 Pacific, on a block now occupied by the Hyatt Regency Hotel. Pass through the square, admiring the public art and the fountain, and continue through Ferry Park to the Embarcadero.

Ferry Building

POINTS OF INTEREST

Slanted Door **1 Ferry Building, 415-861-8032**

Pier 23 Cafe **Pier 23, 415-362-5125**

Fog City Diner **1300 Battery St., 415-982-2000**

Old Ship Saloon **298 Pacific Ave., 415-788-2222**

route Summary

1. Begin at the Ferry Building, at the foot of Market St.
2. Exiting the Ferry Building, turn right onto the Embarcadero, heading north.
3. Walk past Pier 23, cross the Embarcadero, and return down the other side, heading south.
4. Where Battery St. begins, follow it on the left side of the street for less than a block and turn into the park.
5. Follow the trail through the park until it reaches Levi Strauss Plaza.
6. Turn right, into the plaza, and follow the open quad to Sansome St.
7. Turn left onto Sansome St.
8. Turn left on Green St.
9. Turn right on Front St.
10. Turn right on Pacific Ave.
11. Turn left on Battery St.
12. Turn left on Jackson St.
13. Turn left on Front St.
14. Enter Sydney Walton Square, cut through the park toward the exit at the corner of Davis and Jackson streets.
15. Cut through Ferry Park, follow trail back to the Embarcadero.

Sailor's delight—the Old Ship Saloon

Jackson St

Hotaling St

Embarcadero Plaza

Washington St

Merchant St

finish

Merchant St

Embarcadero Center

Davis St

Drumm St

Merchant St

Clay St

Grant Ave

Waverly Pl

Commercial St

Leidesdorff St

Sacramento St

Front St

Sacramento St

Kearny St

Spring St

Halleck St

California St

Davis St

California St

Quincy St

Grant Ave

Pine St

Pine St

Battery St

EMBARCADERO

Beale St

Sacramento St

Belden Pl

Montgomery St

Sansome St

Bush St

Market St

Fremont St

Harlan Pl

Claude Ln

Bush St

Trinity Pl

Sutter St

1st St

Sutter St

Lick Pl

Market St

Stevenson St

Jessie St

Elim St

Mission St

Campton Pl

Post St

MONTGOMERY ST

start

2nd St

Minna St

Natoma St

0   100   200   300 yards

0   100   200   300 meters

3 FINANCIAL DISTRICT: THROUGH THE PILLARS OF CAPITALISM

BOUNDARIES: **Market St., Kearny St., Washington St., Front St.**
DISTANCE: **1¾ miles**
DIFFICULTY: **Easy**
PARKING: **Russ Building Garage, 235 Montgomery St.**
PUBLIC TRANSIT: **Montgomery St. BART station; Muni J, K, L, M, and N trains, F Streetcars, and 5, 6, 9, 21, 31, and 71 Muni buses**

This is where the big wheels turn in San Francisco. Looking much like a short section of Midtown Manhattan or the Loop in Chicago, the Financial District is a grid of canyons formed by the high-rise pillars of capitalism. Buildings bold, stately, and conservative tell the secret that lies at the core of San Francisco's history and character, for while the cultural icons of the city are gold diggers, gays, and hippies, it was the staunch businesses of banking, stock brokering, real estate, and shipping that put the city on the map. Suitably, the Financial District resulted from a frantic scramble for well-positioned real estate. During the Gold Rush, each time valuable bayfront lots were sold, a little more bay was filled, creating new bayfront property. (It was tough luck for the guy with last year's dockside office.)

It's not particularly comforting to consider that skyscrapers and landfill make an unhealthy combination in earthquake country, which is why San Francisco's skyline remained relatively low until quake-resistant steel-frame construction came into vogue. The foundations of the district's skyscrapers stand on pilings driven deep into the earth, and the more modern towers are designed to sway gently in a temblor.

The Financial District may be cold at heart, but during workdays its sidewalks are alive with fast-paced, cell-phone-driven human activity. Restaurants, small museums, and rooftop observatories afford the interloper ample opportunity to see the district from the inside out.

● **Start at the former Crocker Bank Building, now owned by Wells Fargo, at 1 Montgomery St. The curved columned entry makes an effective statement on this prominent corner, but what's really interesting about the building is that it was once** ten stories taller. It was truncated in the mid-1960s to broaden the views from the Wells Fargo tower behind it. The building's much diminished rooftop is an open observatory, so go inside, take the elevator up, and have a look around.

- Follow Montgomery to Sutter and turn left. Half a block up, at No. 130, is the Halladie Building, noted for being among the first glass curtain–wall buildings in the world. Its glass face is supported by a steel frame—a style not at all rare today, but nearly unique in 1917 when it was built. Willis Polk designed it. Note the tastefully curved fire escapes, which enhance the building's looks as well as provide a way out in the event of a blaze.

- At Kearny turn right, cross at Bush and turn right again. At the corner of Belden and Bush, Sam's Grill is a neighborhood institution with a traditional San Francisco menu based on seafood, pasta, and sourdough bread. The interior booths have curtains, for the privacy of patrons who need to hash out a shady deal. It's not romantic, but very cool in its Sam Spade urbanness.

- Head up Belden, a one-block pedestrian alley that's lined with French restaurants. The area, including a block or two of Bush St., is known as the "French Ghetto." During lunch and dinner hours, especially on warm days, the alley is crammed with little tables where off-duty white-collar workers enjoy mussels from Plouf or steak frites from Cafe Bastille.

- At the end of Belden Place, hook left and continue down Kearny, walking in the shadow of the Bank of America Building, which stands 52 stories tall. It was San Francisco's tallest building until the Transamerica Pyramid went up a few years later. Look up from any perspective, and the building's striking sawtooth bays, slicing into the sky, catch and reflect light and color. Wide steps meet a raised plaza with a hulking black sculpture that's broadly referred to as the "Banker's Heart."

- Follow Kearny to Sacramento, turn right, and turn right again at Montgomery. The Wells Fargo History Museum is worth a quick visit to get a rosy perspective on one of the city's biggest and oldest financial institutions. (Wells Fargo opened its first office in San Francisco in 1852.) It won't require more than a few minutes to take an up-close look at the museum's old stagecoach. In addition to banking, Wells Fargo initially ran a network of stages across the Western U.S. until the arrival of the rail-roads. Admission to the museum is free.

● At the corner of Montgomery and California—the geographic epicenter of the Financial District—turn right. The Merchants Exchange Building (465 California St.) was designed by Daniel Burnham and reflects his Chicago School architectural style. It was built in 1903. Enter the building and pass through the long lobby to enter the California Bank Trust, where the glory of the building's maritime past is celebrated with huge murals by Walter Coulter and Nils Hagerup. Architect Julia Morgan kept her offices on the top floor of the building.

● Exit a side door onto tiny Leidesdorff St., a narrow lane that appears determined not to attract attention. Before the 1906 quake, Leidesdorff was known as "Pauper Alley." As wild speculation on silver mining went on elsewhere in the district, Leidesdorff was lined with small-time exchanges where the nearly penni-less could invest a few cents in hopes of turning their luck around. The street apparently had few, if any, rags-to-riches tales.

● Return to California St., and opposite, on the corner of Sansome, you'll spot the impos-ing Bank of California, a monumental, mausoleum-like structure erected in 1908. Step inside and you'll see that the entire building is, essentially, one huge, cavernous room with enough airspace beneath its vaulted ceiling to fly a small airplane, if such a thing were permitted. It's a glorious waste of space for such a high-rent dis-trict. Down in the basement, a small museum (free admission) has a few intriguing items, including gold nug-gets imbedded in chunks of quartz,

Wells Fargo Bank

and some territorial gold coins and shiny ingots from the Gold Rush.

● Turn right at Sansome and right again at Pine. On the opposite corner is the Pacific Stock Exchange. Stockbrokers once worked here, and now that it has become a fitness club they work out here. The building was built in 1915, and apparently the stock market crash necessitated a 1930 remodeling job, with designs by Timothy Pflueger. The stoic sculpted figures on both sides of the broad front stairway are by Ralph Stackpole, who in the early 20th century was a central figure in the city's art scene. A side entrance on Sansome leads to the private City Club, in which a two-story mural by Diego Rivera graces a stairwell, which can be seen by nonmembers on a guided tour (call 415-648-7198).

● Turn left at Montgomery, onto a block dominated by two handsome landmarks. The Russ Building, at No. 235, was the city's tallest for several decades after it was built in 1928. Opposite, at No. 220, the Mills Building is the city's archetypal Chicago-style office building. A Daniel Burnham–John Wellborn Root collaboration, it was built in 1892 and survived the '06 catastrophe, though extensive remodeling was required. It was the first all-steel frame structure in the city.

Back Story: Frank Chu

While walking along Montgomery St., you might run into Frank Chu, a man who always has something on his mind and puts it on a sign, which he carries up and down the street nearly every day. He's been walking this beat, sharing his cryptic views, since 1996. For years, Chu advocated impeaching President Bill Clinton, even after Clinton was no longer president. Locals have taken an interest in this eccentric character, mostly because the Frank Chu message turns out to be as bizarre and intricately worked out as you might imagine. Many of Chu's signs refer to the "12 Galaxies," which he claims influenced Clinton to commit treason. He also holds Clinton responsible for not paying Chu for appearing in a reality TV show. Adidas and Quiznos have paid to put advertising on his signs, and the defunct 12 Galaxies nightclub in the Mission District, whose name was inspired by Chu, let him drink at the bar for free. Amid the suited desk jockeys of the Financial District, Frank Chu stands out as an individual who has found an entirely unique way to make a living.

- At Sutter turn left. At the corner of Sutter and Sansome is the Citicorp Center, which was built in 1910 and gutted in 1984, reducing it to an atrium for a new adjacent tower. The atrium is open to the public during business hours. Inside, beyond the cafe tables and fountain, you'll spot the *Star Girl* statue. She's a sight for sore eyes, a replica of a parapet ornament from the Panama Pacific Exposition, which took place in the Marina District in 1914.

- Turn left onto Market St., and to your left is the green-tinted Crown-Zellerbach Building, a glass-curtain beauty from 1959. Unlike nearly every other building in the cramped Financial District, the Crown-Zellerbach is set off the street, with paved grounds surrounding it.

- Turn left at Battery and left again at Bush, where two contrasting structures stand side-by-side. The elegant Shell Building, at 100 Bush, is a sleek skyscraper clad in terra-cotta. It dwarfs its neighbor, the pencil-thin Heineman Building, at No. 130. Designed by George Applegarth, and built in 1910, the Heineman Building makes the fullest use of its slender, 20-foot lot. Its bay façade protrudes beyond the plane of the adjacent buildings, and its cornice actually overlaps them.

- Loop around to California St. via Sansome, Pine, and Battery. At 240 California St, half a block off Battery, Tadich Grill is a revered establishment. It can claim to be the oldest restaurant in the city, having opened in 1849. It has occupied its present site since the late 1960s, and it has the atmosphere of a much older place because the previous location, on Clay St., was stripped, moved, and reassembled here. Busy as ever, Tadich continues to please diners hankering for traditional Frisco dishes such as sand dabs, seafood cioppino, and Dungeness crab cakes.

- At Front St. turn left and head into the Embarcadero Center. This four-tower complex, with a shopping center on the bottom two floors and offices above, was loosely modeled on New York's Rockefeller Center. Walk up the winding stairs to the second level and follow the foot bridge that crosses over Battery St. As you cross you'll get a good vantage of the Old Federal Reserve Building, an imposing neo-Classical structure built in 1924. You can walk through the lobby, graced by a Jules Guerin mural.

● Follow Clay St. to Montgomery and the Transamerica Building, which for obvious reasons is commonly known as the Transamerica Pyramid. Standing 853 feet, it is the tallest building in San Francisco. Initially after it was completed in 1972 it was unpopular, mostly for being so conspicuous. Some detractors needled architect William Pereira by calling it "Pereira's Prick." By now, it is difficult to imagine San Francisco's skyline without the pyramid's pointed top. Walk around the building, and on the Washington St. side you'll find an entrance to Redwood Park, a fine spot to end this tour amidst the tallest trees and the tallest building.

POINTS OF INTEREST

Sam's Grill 374 Bush St., 415-421-0594

Plouf 40 Belden Place, 415-986-6491

Cafe Bastille 22 Belden Place, 415-986-5673

Wells Fargo History Museum 420 Montgomery St., 415-396-2619

The City Club of San Francisco 155 Sansome St., 415-362-2480

Tadich Grill 240 California St., 415-391-1849

route summary

1. Start at the corner of Montgomery and Market and head north, into the Financial District.
2. Turn left at Sutter St.
3. Turn right at Kearny St.
4. Cross Bush St., turn right, and then left onto Belden Place.
5. Turn left on Pine St.
6. Continue on Kearny to Sacramento St. and turn right.
7. Turn right at Montgomery St.
8. Turn left at California St.
9. Turn right at Sansome St.
10. Turn right at Pine St.
11. Turn left at Montgomery St.
12. Turn left at Sutter St.
13. Head east on Market St.
14. Turn left at Battery St.
15. Turn left at Bush St.
16. Turn right at Sansome St.
17. Turn right at Pine St.
18. Turn left at Battery St.
19. Turn right at California St.
20. Turn left at Front St.
21. At the Embarcadero, go up winding stairs beneath the pedestrian overpass.
22. On the second level cross the pedestrian overpass, follow it past Battery and down ramp.
23. Turn right at Sansome St.
24. Turn left at Clay St.
25. Turn right at Montgomery St.
26. Turn right at Washington St.
27. Enter Redwood Park.

Federal Reserve Building

Pine St

Stockton St

WALK 4 UNION SQUARE

Bush St

Kearny St

Claude Ln

Powell St

Joice St

Bush St

Taylor St

Mason St

Sutter St

Campton Pl

Grant Ave

Sutter St

Post St

Post St

Cosmo Pl

Union Square

Maiden Ln

Geary St

Geary St

Grant Ave

Market St

3rd St

Shannon St

finish

Powell St

Stockton St

O'Farrell St

Taylor St

Ellis St

Ellis St

start

Market St

4th St

Yerba
Buena
Gardens

Jones St

Mason St

POWELL ST

Westfield
San Francisco
Centre

Metreon

Eddy St

5th St

Mission St

Moscone West

| 0 | 100 | 200 | 300 yards |
| 0 | 100 | 200 | 300 meters |

4 UNION SQUARE: MINING THE COMMERCIAL MOTHER LODE

BOUNDARIES: **Market St., Taylor St., Bush St., Grant Ave.**
DISTANCE: **1½ miles**
DIFFICULTY: **Moderately easy (one hill, some stairs)**
PARKING: **Off-street parking is available at the Fifth and Mission St. Garage, a block south of the start of this tour.**
PUBLIC TRANSIT: **Powell St. BART station; underground Muni light rail, streetcars, and 5, 6, 9, 21, 31, and 71 Muni buses all stop at the starting point for this tour. So do Powell St. cable cars.**

With its historic buildings, showpiece retail stores, fine restaurants, theaters, hotels, billboards clamoring for rooftop exposure, and converging public transit lines, Union Square has all the hallmarks of a commercial and cultural hub. It's a central crossroads that has a way of drawing people and traffic through it. Day and night, the area buzzes with cars and buses starting and stopping at traffic lights, the groaning of cable car brakes, the repertoire of street corner singers, the purposeful clicking of high heel shoes, and the toot of whistles blown by hotel doormen hailing cabs. This tour will range a bit freely, proceeding from Market St. to Union Square itself in the least direct route possible without leaving the neighborhood.

- Start at the Powell St. cable car turnaround, on the corner of Market and Powell. If it's the summer tourist season, a hundred or more people will be lined up here for a ride on the historic cable cars, and a multitude of street performers will be vying for their attention and spare change. Don't get in line, but wait for a cable car to come along, and watch how it is rolled onto the circular platform, then rotated 180 degrees, all by hand, as it has been done for over 130 years.

- Overlooking the cable car turnaround is the staunch and impressive Flood Building, with a huge Gap flagship store occupying the ground floor. The building is a quake survivor. It was designed by Albert Pissis and built in 1904. Dashiell Hammett worked upstairs for the Pinkerton Agency during the early 1920s, a few years before he published the novels that would make him a famous crime fiction writer. Walk along

Powell St., below the block-long Flood Building, and hook right on Ellis St. Half a block up you'll spot John's Grill, which has been operating since 1908. Hammett reputedly dined at John's frequently, and even mentioned the place in his best novel, *The Maltese Falcon*.

● Return to Powell and turn right. The street is a disorganized mélange of shops and hotels geared to tourists and passers-through. In the mix are some age-old establishments that seem to hang on despite the changing vibe of the neighborhood. These blocks of Powell St. not so long ago had some of the Tenderloin's flophouse atmosphere. Tad's Steaks, with its excellent gaudy sign looking like a holdover from the vaudeville era, still purveys shoeleather cuts, charbroiled and served over the counter. At Powell and O'Farrell, Marquard's Little Cigar Store closed a few years back but its stylish curved sign, wrapping around the corner, remains. Some San Franciscans lamented the closing of the shop, but it turns out they really only thought they'd miss the sign.

Near the corner of Geary, the Gold Dust Lounge keeps alcoholic hours (opening at 7 a.m.) and features a live band nightly. Until recently, the music of choice here was Dixieland, or the final traces of a long-dead form. San Francisco was way into Dixieland long after New York went bop and L.A. went cool. It was the hokey jazz of strumming banjos and swooning trombones, performed by musicians in straw boaters and shirtsleeve garters, which perhaps represented some lost connection to the Barbary Coast. The Gold Dust was the music's last gasp, and without it the place is less interesting.

● Turn left on Geary, and more roughs appear amidst the diamonds. Lefty O'Doul's is named for a nearly forgotten baseball hero who won the National League batting title in 1929, finishing just two-points shy of a .400 average. He led the league again three seasons later. The bar's a great spot for perusing local sports memorabilia, and the stools have baseball bats for legs. It's also a bustling hofbrau where the hot open-faced turkey sandwich is a fine mess to get yourself into. At night someone tinkles the ivories (or sets up a cheesy synthesizer on top of the piano) and croons familiar chestnuts.

At the corner of Geary and Mason stands the Pinecrest Diner, a 24-hour eatery that's been slinging the neighborhood's hash since 1969. Looks like it's been here longer than that. It's the no-nonsense, Hopper painting atmosphere—not the food—

that draws people. The place is genuinely hard-boiled, and a little tragic. In 1997, a grill cook shot and killed a waitress in the restaurant.

● The Pinecrest inadvertently ushers us into the Theater District, with two landmark stages standing side-by-side on the block. The Geary Theater opened in 1909 and is now home of the highly respected American Conservatory Theater. The building is a beauty clad in terra-cotta tiles, many of them shaped like fruit. To the right of the front entrance a traditional shoeshine stand operates during the business week. The Geary is best admired from across the street, where you can see the entire building. Next door, the Curran was built in 1922, and though it's not bearing fruit, it and the Geary make a very compatible pair. Theaters small and large are scattered all throughout the neighborhood.

● At the end of the block stands the Clift Hotel, which through a recent remodel has successfully reentered the ranks of the city's most sophisticated hostelries. The Clift always had the Redwood Room, a gorgeous, clubby old watering hole, and those in the know long appreciated their martinis here. The joint's fashionable now, with a velvet rope and a bouncer to maintain order on Friday and Saturday nights. On quieter weeknights it is still possible to enjoy a relaxed drink here amid early-20th-century splendor.

Across from the Clift is another pompous old hotel, the Monaco, which has retained much of its steamship-era pizzazz. You need only step into the hotel's restaurant, the Grand Cafe, to get an idea of how much pampering goes on here. In a former ballroom, the Grand makes a convincing argument that size matters. There's plenty of room for left-handers at the tables here,

The Flood Building

and it probably takes two waiters to change the light bulbs—one to screw in the bulb, one to hold the ladder. It's a good spot for lunch, if eating is in your plans.

● Turn right at Taylor. Halfway up the block look for tiny Isadora Duncan Lane, a dead-end alley that rarely benefits from direct sunlight. A monkey could swing from the fire escapes on one side to the fire escapes on the other side. Named for the legendary dancer who was born within a block of here, it is a model for how all dead-end alleys ought to look.

The stately ivy-covered red-brick fortress on the corner of Taylor and Post is home of the exclusive Bohemian Club. The name was once somewhat appropriate, for when it was founded, in 1872, the club's members were writers, poets, newspaper reporters, and artists. By 1900, however, the club was dominated by businessmen and social elites. All men, of course, and all white. The club hasn't changed much (it's now about 2 percent non-white). U.S. presidents have attended the club's annual summer fetes, which are held two hours north of the city in the Bohemian Grove. George W. Bush and Dick Cheney had a powwow at the Grove in 2000, which supposedly resulted in Cheney joining the Republican ticket. A plaque on the side of the club has a bas relief owl on a branch, along with the words "Weaving spiders come not here"—meaning what? No knitting widows allowed? The vast majority of San Franciscans regard the Bohemian Club with distrust and disdain.

● Turn right on Post and cross Mason. On the north side of the street is Farallon, one of the city's best seafood restaurants. Step inside for a look at the outlandish underwater decor, a Jules Verne fantasy, with illuminated jellyfish hanging from the ceiling.

● At Powell turn left. Two local landmarks face off on this block. On the west side is humble Sears' Fine Foods, known the world over for its dollar-sized pancakes. It was opened in 1938 by Ben Sears. Nearly every reference to Sears mentions he was a retired circus clown, so let's not overlook that important detail. Opposite is the Sir Francis Drake Hotel. Cross at Sutter and backtrack to the hotel's front entrance and be sure to smile at the Beefeater doorman on your way in. Inside, examine the magnificent staircase with its intricate cast-iron rail, and gape at the molded plaster ceiling above. Then duck downstairs, where an elevator can take you to the Starlight Room, a swanky top-floor nightclub surrounded by plate-glass windows. Back at the bottom floor, exit the Drake through the side exit, onto Sutter St., cross at the light and turn right.

● The office tower at 450 Sutter is mostly populated by doctors and dentists, but the building is a pure flight of fancy. It was designed by Timothy Pflueger, who also designed the magnificent Castro Theatre and the Paramount Theatre in Oakland. The lobby at 450 Sutter looks like a set for a never-made Cecil B. DeMille epic about the Mayan empire. It's well worth going in for a look-see. From the sidewalk the tower's jagged columns of bay windows are fine to look at too.

● At Stockton turn left and you're soon facing the southern end of the Stockton Tunnel. The entry looks inviting, despite the sign that says QUIET IN TUNNEL, but it's just your usual tunnel, dank and dimly lit. Immediately within, a foul-smelling flight of steps leads up to Bush St., which is where we're headed.

● The Tunnel Top bar, a refurbished dive that's kind of hip now, welcomes you to Bush St. If you're in a drinking mood, have one of the bar's signature mojitos. Just past the Tunnel Top, on a wall flanking narrow Burritt Alley, a plaque notes that Sam Spade's partner, Miles Archer, was "done in" on this spot by Brigid O'Shaughnessy. It's great to see completely fictional events getting historic markers. You can walk away with this lesson: always cross-check anything you've read on a plaque. On the other side of the street, another alley is named for Hammett.

● Now turn around and walk down Bush. Elegant Notre Dame des Victoires, a Catholic church, stands at No. 566. It was originally built in 1855, then rebuilt after the '06 quake. Inside the church, the grand pipe organ is worthy of landmark status, having been built in 1915 by the Johnston Organ and Piano Manufacturing Company. It is renowned for its beautiful tone, which you may hear if you attend a Saturday Vigil, with an organist accompanying a cantor, at 5:15 p.m.

● At Grant turn right, stopping for a quick look at the groovy Hotel Triton, a boutique hostelry that trades on the city's countercultural heritage. For the heck of it ask to see a room and you might be shown the Carlos Santana or Jerry Garcia suites (supposedly with design input from these guys) or a tiny "zen den."

● The southeast corner of Grant and Sutter is dominated by the historic White House department store, which closed its doors years ago. The building is now occupied by Banana Republic. It was designed, with Federalist overtones, by Albert Pissis, and built in 1908.

● Turn right onto slender Maiden Lane, a street that had its name changed in order to obscure a shameful past. Before the '06 quake the street, then called Morton St., was known as one of the city's dreariest hubs of prostitution. Low-life cribs lined both sides of the street. It's much calmer and more respectable now. All there is to see is the Xanadu Gallery, a store that sells fine artifacts and folk art from exotic far-off lands. The building is a Frank Lloyd Wright design built in 1949, and its spiral ramp is often cited as a warm-up for Wright's more accomplished Guggenheim Museum in New York.

● Maiden Lane ends at Union Square. Turn left, walk to the corner of Geary and enter the Neiman Marcus department store. Immediately within, stare up at the great rotunda, with its stained glass mosaic of a ship. It's all that remains of the old City of Paris department store that formerly stood on this corner. The rest of the building was demolished and replaced by the current modern structure in the early 1980s. You can take an elevator to the top floor for a closer look at the glass, or back out now before someone sprays perfume on you.

● Cross to the square. It was part of the original city plans of 1850, and became a more prominent address as the city expanded south from Portsmouth Square. It gained its name during the Civil War. The Dewey Monument, rising like a pin from the square's center, commemorates a victory in the Spanish-American War. A parking structure—meant to double as a bomb shelter—was dug beneath the square during World War II. The square acquired its current Italian piazza styling in a dot-com-era overhaul, and it's a good spot to stop for an outdoor coffee or to see occasional midday music performances. The surrounding cityscape of department stores, billboards, and the awesome Westin St. Francis Hotel makes this a pleasant urban space. You're seeing the St. Francis from its most flattering vantage point.

The St. Francis was built in 1904, and it was gutted by the fire of '06 and rebuilt a year later. It's the grand dame of Union Square, but it hasn't escaped controversy over the years. In 1921 comic actor Fatty Arbuckle rented a suite of rooms and threw the party that ended with the gruesome death of a young actress, Virginia Rappe. Arbuckle was tried for rape and murder, but he wasn't convicted. The scandal nevertheless diminished his comic appeal and put an end to his career. President Gerald Ford was shot at by Sarah Jane Moore in front of the hotel in 1975. She missed, went to jail, escaped, was recaptured, and was paroled in 2007, almost exactly a year after Ford had died of natural causes.

● Enter the St. Francis' main lobby and look for the elevators. The hotel's modern high-rise annex was built in the early 1970s, with high-speed glass elevators shooting skyward along the east side of the building. For kicks, end this tour with a ride up to the top and you'll enjoy a spectacular view as well as the sensation of leaving your stomach two or three floors beneath you.

POINTS OF INTEREST

John's Grill 63 Ellis Street, 415-986-0069

Tad's Steaks 120 Powell St., 415-982-1718

Gold Dust Lounge 247 Powell St., 415-397-1695

Lefty O'Doul's 333 Geary St., 415-982-8900

Pinecrest Diner 401 Geary St., 415-885-6407

Grand Cafe 501 Geary St., 415-292-0101

Farallon 450 Post St., 415-956-6969

Sears' Fine Foods 439 Powell St., 415-986-0700

Starlight Room 450 Powell St., 415-395-8595

Tunnel Top 601 Bush St., 415-986-8900

Notre Dame des Victoires 566 Bush St., 415-397-0113

Hotel Triton 324 Grant Ave., 415-394-0500

Westin St. Francis Hotel 335 Powell St., 415-397-7000

route summary

1.   Start at the corner of Powell and Market streets and head up Powell.

2.   Turn right on Ellis St., walk half a block up, then return to Powell.

3.   Turn right on Powell St.

4.   Turn left on Geary St.

5.   Turn right on Taylor St.

6.   Turn right on Post St.

7.   Turn left on Powell St.

8.   Turn right on Sutter St.

9.   Turn left on Stockton St.

10.   At the entrance to the Stockton Tunnel,
      walk up the stairs to Bush St.

11.   Head west on Bush St. half a block to Burritt Alley.

12.   Turn around and head east on Bush St.

13.   Turn right on Grant Ave.

14.   Turn right on Maiden Lane.

15.   Turn left on Stockton St.

16.   Cross to Union Square.

17.   Cross Powell St. to the Westin St. Francis Hotel.

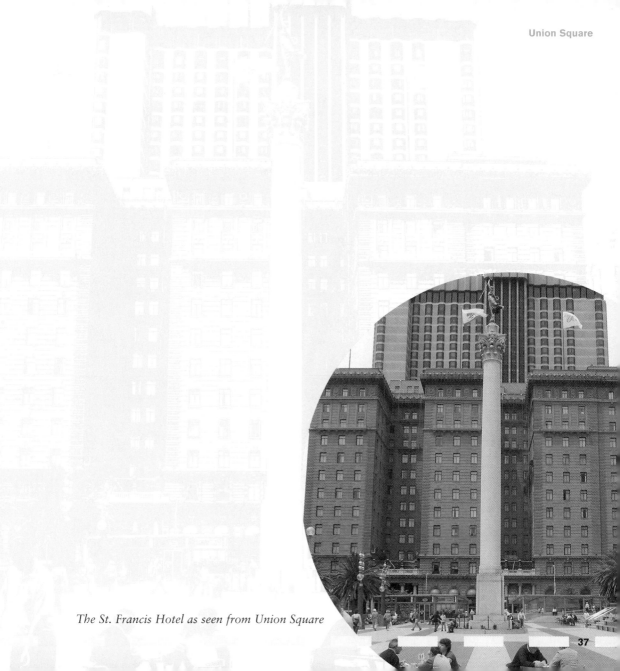

The St. Francis Hotel as seen from Union Square

start

finish

Vallejo St

Broadway

Broadway

Pacific Ave

Columbus Ave

Pacific Ave

Montgomery St

Gold St

Sansome St

Hotaling St

Washington St

John St

Trenton St

Stone St

Stockton St

Ross Alley

Jackson St

Grant Ave

Waverly Pl

Merchant St

Clay St

Commercial St

Mason St

Washington St

Codman Pl

Wetmore St

Sacramento St

Clay St

Spring St

Kearny St

Leidesdorff St

California St

Powell St

Joice St

Stockton St

Grant Ave

Quincy St

Kearny St

St George Aly

Belden Pl

Montgomery St

Petrarch Pl

California St

Pine St

Pine St

Bush St

Trinity Pl

Pine St

Bush St

Harlan Pl

0   100   200   300 yards

0   100   200   300 meters

5 CHINATOWN: THE Far EAST OF THE WEST COAST

BOUNDARIES: **Broadway, Stockton St., Bush St., Grant Ave.**
DISTANCE: **1¾ miles**
DIFFICULTY: **Moderately easy (mild hills)**
PARKING: **Off street parking is available on Vallejo St., between Powell and Stockton (one block from the starting point for this tour)**
PUBLIC TRANSIT: **30, 45 Muni buses**

San Francisco has a Chinatown to rival any city's Chinatown, and like many Chinatowns, San Francisco's has an air of inauthenticity. Many of the buildings here reflect naive American notions of what Eastern architecture ought to look like, with shop fronts resembling pagodas painted in spectacular, often garish colors. Even the lamp posts, fire hydrants, and telephone booths have a kitschy, orientalist look to them. But comparisons to Disneyland don't tell the entire story. In the wake of the '06 quake, men of overwhelming influence, including former mayor James Phelan, wanted to move Chinatown to remote Hunters Point. Chinese businessmen preempted that campaign by rebuilding quickly with over-the-top, undeniably Chinese styles of architecture. Thanks to their efforts, Chinatown stayed put, and to this day it remains one of San Francisco's most vibrant and exciting neighborhoods. Its sidewalks are packed shoulder-to-shoulder with locals every day of the year, and all manner of goods literally spill out of the shops. At night, the district's commercial streets become a relatively subdued and atmospheric constellation of neon. This walk follows the main thoroughfares, Stockton St. and Grant Ave., with frequent detours through mysterious alleys smelling of cabbage and into clamorous dim sum parlors where you'd hardly know you were still in North America.

● A daytime visit to Chinatown should include a stop for dim sum, and since Gold Mountain, at 644 Broadway, is the quintessential dim sum restaurant, it makes a good place to start. Show up around 11 a.m. and you'll find yourself in a crowded hall alive with chatter, mostly in Cantonese. A fleet of carts rolls through the aisles bearing steaming hot morsels such as silky shrimp crepes, deep-fried shrimp balls, flaky xiu mai, and piping hot pots of congee (rice porridge). Thus fortified, hit the streets and work it off.

● Head up Broadway and turn left onto Stockton St. This is the district's "real" side, unadorned and untouristy, and fulfilling most of the neighborhood's day-to-day requirements. Along Stockton, in stores dealing in miscellaneous household goods, the aisles are choked with plastic buckets, dayglo brooms, teapots, soup bowls, meat cleavers, chopsticks, bulky flesh-toned bras, and tiny folding chairs for children. There are numerous jewelry shops, some with signs advertising gold bullion, and not quite as many hair salons. Bakeries sell moon cakes, wedding cakes, and little round balls filled with mung bean paste. Produce shops can hardly contain all that they offer: Asian pears, jujubes, lychees, longans, boiled peanuts, bok choi, water chestnuts, Chinese broccoli, yams, tangelos, and taro root. Some shops specialize in anything that has had the life dried out of it: dried shrimp, dried squid, dried oysters, countless varieties of mushrooms, and ginseng by the barrel. Roasted ducks and chickens hang in windows. Entire pigs, ghostly white, hang on meat hooks beyond side doors left wide open to the street. The shop at 1135 Stockton, between Pacific and Jackson, is a dim, damp hall that lures in its clientele with tanks filled with catatonic rock fish, tubs of live frogs that aren't hopping away, and snails packed on ice. Farther in, glass cases display the internal organs of pigs and cows, and still deeper a little shop within the larger shop stocks chickens and pigeons kept in cages. Stroll the next few blocks and duck into shops that intrigue you. Stockton is also the street on which you're most likely to be nudged out of an old lady's way, so watch your step.

● Turn right at Clay. Half a block up, the Chinese Historical Society of America operates a museum (noon to 5 p.m. Tuesday through Friday) in a former YWCA building. The permanent collection is modest, but special exhibits focusing on Chinese life in California from the Gold Rush to the present are generally worth a look. Admission is $3.

● Return to Stockton and turn right. The building at No. 843 is home of the Consolidated Benevolent Association, also known as the "Chinese Six Companies." The Six Companies is far more than a family association or social aid club. It is a conglomeration of such community groups that started forming in the late 19th century, at a time when Chinatown society was severely constrained by laws limiting their movements within the broader society and continually disrupted by ongoing tong wars between rival criminal gangs. The Six Companies became for a time the most powerful Chinese American political organization in the country. The Six Companies remains highly influential in San Francisco's Chinese community today.

● Across the street, at No. 836, is Sun Yat-Sen Memorial Hall, and next door to that is the local Kuomintang headquarters. KMT, the Chinese Nationalist Party, vied for control of mainland China from 1912 until the Communist victory in 1949, and then dominated Taiwanese politics for most of the 20th century. It has historically drawn wide support from San Francisco's Chinese community.

● Turn left onto Sacramento, and at Waverly Place stop in at the Clarion Music Center, a shop that sells beautiful instruments used in the traditional music of China. There's a room devoted to high-quality gongs of all sizes and timbres, and even a full-length lion dance costume, but the shop's primary emphasis is on the erhu, the two-string spike fiddle played so mournfully in some of the neighborhood's alleys. If you're in a buying mood, rest assured you can also learn to play the instrument here.

● Walk the two-block length of Waverly, a narrow road that's not quite small enough to be considered an alley. In the late 19th century it was lined with barber shops, and because the price of a trim was 15 cents, Waverly was known as "15 Cent Street." There's still a solitary barber shop, called Li Ly's Hair Salon, that charges $5 for a cut. Waverly is a colorful street, with many painted balconies and decorative tiles on the facades of the buildings. Signs over the doorways indicate numerous family associations are based here, and there are a smattering of Buddhist temples hidden away on some of the top floors. One, Tin How Temple, is open to visitors

Pagoda-style architecture

(10 a.m.–4 p.m.). It's well worth the schlep up three flights of stairs for what feels like a privileged behind-the-scenes look into this otherwise private neighborhood. The presentation is minimal but welcoming. Volunteers will deliver a prepared narration to explain the altar and the joss sticks spiraling overhead.

- Where Waverly meets Washington, take a quick right to Sam Wo Restaurant, where the woeful food is legendary. Years ago, this place was popular simply because its head waiter, who called himself Edsel Ford, was so comically rude to the patrons. Jack Kerouac supposedly learned to use chopsticks here while chomping on chow mein with his friend, the poet Gary Snyder. Sam Wo's is still worth the resulting heartburn for the nonpareil atmosphere—guests pass through the kitchen, up twisting narrow stairs, into cramped unadorned dining rooms, where they are greeted by a mildly rude waiter (following in the late Mr. Ford's footsteps). Meals are shuttled up from the kitchen in a rickety old dumbwaiter.

- Backtrack up Washington, cross the street, and head up Ross Alley, a mysterious passageway known in the 19th century as the "Street of the Gamblers" because so many gambling joints were located here. Down near the end of the block, beneath the nearly continuous canopy of fire escapes, slip into the Golden Gate Fortune Cookie Company where you can see how fortune cookies are made. The cast-iron machinery in the shop looks like it was built in the age of steam engines, and the workers who fold the still hot cookies by hand, after first slipping the fortunes in, are quick and deft. Someone will stop and sell you a bag of fresh cookies if you like, but the staff are generally too busy to field questions. A couple of doors down, Jun Yu's Barber Shop is easily passed unnoticed, but be sure to pause for a peek inside. It's the world's smallest, most cluttered barbershop, with barely room for a chair and a barber to move in. When business is slow the barber passes the time in front of his shop, reading the paper or bowing his erhu fiddle. You'll notice 4-by-6-inch snaps of celebrities like Matt Dillon and Michael Douglas in the shop window. Over the years the place has attracted the attention of Hollywood location scouts, and a number of films have included scenes shot here. The evidence—more snaps, and excerpts on YouTube—suggests singer Tom Waits was the only celeb to actually get his ears lowered here.

- At Jackson turn right, and at Grant Ave. turn right again. On this block, you'll spot two old drinking taverns, the garish Li Po (named for a poet) and the more somnolent Buddha Bar (named for a god). Both places look like World War II shore-leave saloons and are good for a quiet cold one in the afternoon.

- Just off Grant at 743 Washington, the United Commercial Bank occupies a building, built after the 1906 quake, that is worthy of a movie set. It was once the Chinese Telephone Exchange. In order to handle the complex mix of cultures and languages in Chinatown, the operators who worked the exchange were fluent in five Chinese dialects in addition to English. The building's interior was remodeled to look more like a bank, but from the street it retains its pseudo pagoda stature.

- Return to Grant and halfway down the block you'll reach the Empress of China, a posh restaurant that had its heyday in the middle of the 20th century. Enter the lobby (the actual dining room is on the top floor) for a look at the celebrity snaps posted near the elevator. You'll see some comical surprises, including Raymond Burr from his *Ironside* period and a rather exuberant Jayne Mansfield. Loads of others.

- For eight blocks Grant Ave., Chinatown's touristy main drag, is crammed with shops selling kitschy curios. Here you'll find paper lanterns, calligraphy scrolls, silk pajamas, silk scarves, black canvas slippers, jade Buddhas, red-lacquered Buddhas, ceramic Buddhas, ceramic dragons, ceramic pigs emblazoned with floral patterns, bobble-headed cats that wave one paw, Obama bobble-heads, fancy kites, license plates and street signs with popular children's names on them, pink conical hats, jewelry, antiques, elephant tusks intricately carved to look like miniature shangri-las, T-shirts that say "got dim sum?", shot glasses, swords, giant vases, discount luggage, dainty parasols, life-sized statues of Indians shooting bows and arrows, and life-sized stat-ues of horses rearing on hind legs, should you need anything like that. Needless to say, many of the shops are worth picking through. Canton Bazaar, to single out just one, sells everything from chopsticks to "sensual" statues that are displayed behind a glass case. At least step in to admire the lovely lacquered painting, two-stories tall, that hangs in the south stairwell. When asked, the woman behind the counter said she had no idea who painted it, and neither did her boss, but it's an impressive sight. A couple blocks up, Red Blossom Tea Company sells fine teas and beautiful Yixing tea pots, fashioned by hand in the Sung Dynasty style of a millennium ago. Closer to Broadway, Golden Gate Bakery is a busy little shop that sells delicate custard-filled pastries, which often attract lines out the door.

● The intersection of Grant and California is a pivotal crossroads in Chinatown, with several landmark buildings, including the first two fake pagodas to go up after the '06 quake. The intersection is flanked by the exotic Sing Fat Building, at 717 California St., which went up in 1907 and the Sing Chong Building, at 601 Grant, which went up a year later. Also at this intersection stands Old St. Mary's, a quake survivor that dates all the way back to 1853. This old church has seen it all, which adds some weight to the sign below the clock, which quotes Ecclesiastes: SON, OBSERVE THE TIME AND FLY FROM EVIL.

● Cross California, turn left, and make a quick right at Quincy St., into St. Mary's Square. The park is a hidden sanctuary amid the neighborhood's hustle and bustle. Often you'll encounter locals doing their tai chi exercises here. At the center of the square, a statue of Sun Yat-Sen, looking a little like the Tin Man in *The Wizard of Oz,* is the work of sculptor Beniamino Bufano.

● At Pine, turn right, which gets you back to Grant. Follow it all the way to the Chinatown Gate, at Bush St., and you'll have seen quite a lot of Chinatown. The neighborhood warrants further exploration, so you may want to wander back through all the streets we haven't hit on this tour.

POINTS OF INTEREST

Gold Mountain 644 Broadway, 415-296-7733

The Chinese Historical Society of America 965 Clay St., 415-391-1188

Clarion Music Center 816 Sacramento St., 415-391-1317

Sam Wo Restaurant 813 Washington St., 415-982-0596

Golden Gate Fortune Cookie Company 56 Ross Alley, 415-781-3956

Li Po 916 Grant Ave., 415-982-0072

Buddha Bar 901 Grant Ave., 415-362-1792

United Commercial Bank (Old Chinese Telephone Exchange) 743 Washington St.

Canton Bazaar 616 Grant Ave., 415-362-5750

Red Blossom Tea Company 831 Grant Ave., 415-395-0868

Golden Gate Bakery 1029 Grant Ave., 415-781-2627

route summary

1. Start at Gold Mountain, on Broadway just above Columbus St.
2. Turn left at Stockton St.
3. Turn right at Clay St.
4. Return to Stockton and turn right.
5. Turn left at Sacramento St.
6. Turn left at Waverly Place.
7. Turn right briefly onto Washington St. (for Sam Wo's), then cross and head up Ross Alley.
8. Turn right at Jackson St.
9. Turn right on Grant Ave.
10. Turn right at California St.
11. Turn right at Quincy St., leading into St. Mary's Square.
12. Turn right at Pine St.
13. Turn left at Grant Ave.
14. End at Bush St. at the Chinatown Gate.

Sun Yat-Sen by Beniamino Bufano

Vallejo St

Grant Ave

Fresno St

Romolo Pl

Kearny St

Montgomery St

Bartol St

Broadway

Sansome St

Osgood Pl

Battery St

finish

Broadway

Columbus Ave

Pacific Ave

Gold St

Jackson St

Columbus Ave

Beckett St

Hotaling St

Sansome St

Custom House Pl

Jackson St

Wentworth Pl

Kearny St

Gibb St

Grant Ave

Ross Alley

Washington St

Washington St

Merchant St

Merchant St

Montgomery St

start

Portsmouth Square

Walter Lum Pl

Waverly Pl

Spofford St

Clay St

Clay St

Clay St

| 0 | 50 | 100 | 150 yards |

| 0 | 50 | 100 | 150 meters |

6   Jackson Square: Time Traveling Through the Barbary Coast

BOUNDARIES: **Washington St., Kearny St., Sansome St., Broadway**
DISTANCE: **¾ mile**
DIFFICULTY: **Easy**
PARKING: **A public parking lot is hidden beneath Portsmouth Square**
PUBLIC TRANSIT: **1, 8X Muni buses**

There is little disputing that San Francisco got off to a spectacular start. By all accounts, the city was thrown up with the purposeful chaos of a carnival pulling into town in the dark of night. For decades the atmosphere in many parts of town pulsed with a hell's a-poppin' spirit. The area between the main plaza and the wharves managed to distinguish itself as particularly rough, and became known as the Barbary Coast.

The name suggested a likeness to the pirate-infested coast of North Africa, where European sailors risked being captured and enslaved on corsair galleys. The district functioned like an angler fish preying upon sin-seeking sailors. For its lure it had block after block of gambling dens, whorehouses, music halls, saloons, and boardinghouses. Serious consequences awaited those who were outsmarted here. The neighborhood was rife with swindlers and shanghai-ers. For the unwary miner or shore-leave sailor, the path of least resistance generally led to a knock-out blow in the back room of a saloon.

The district began to form with the arrival of the first Forty-niners and thrived until the devastating quake and fire of 1906. Ironically, the buildings in this haven of heathens were largely spared by that catastrophe. Some buildings were torn down later, but the district is now listed on the National Register and protected. Most of Pacific St., popularly known as "Terrific Street" when it was the main stem of the Barbary Coast, is now a quiet row of distinguished antique dealers and architectural firms.

● **Start in Portsmouth Square, which during the Gold Rush was the city's main plaza. City Hall stood on Kearny St. from 1852 to 1895. It occupied the former Jenny Lind Theater, so named in honor of the "Swedish Nightingale," who never performed in**

San Francisco. Next door was a grand gambling hall called El Dorado. The legendary Bella Union, most popular of the city's music halls, stood on Washington St., just above Kearny. The square itself was a barren patch of earth with criss-crossing footpaths converging in the middle. This is where important things happened in early San Francisco. In July 1846, the Stars and Stripes were raised here by Captain John B. Montgomery, formally claiming the settlement of Yerba Buena for the U.S. (The town was renamed San Francisco a year later.) A plaque in the square commemorates the event. The square soon acquired the name of Montgomery's ship, the USS *Portsmouth*. Another monument, featuring a cast bronze ship, commemorates a couple of visits by Robert Louis Stevenson, author of the classic tale *Treasure Island*. Having spent a few months in San Francisco in 1879, Stevenson returned in 1888 with his new wife, Fanny. From here they embarked on the extended sea voyage that would end with the author's death in Samoa, six years later. Now firmly part of Chinatown, Portsmouth Square looks nothing like it would have before 1906, but it is as vital as ever. It still attracts gamblers—on pretty much any day of the week you'll spot men gathered around park benches playing fevered games of cards.

Follow Washington St. in the direction of the bay, cross Columbus Ave., and you're entering the Jackson Square Historic District. Most of the brick structures here date to the 1850s and '60s, when this area was the city's exciting and dangerous nightlife zone.

The Transamerica Pyramid (which we examined in the Financial District walk) stands on a historic site, that of the legendary Montgomery Block, commonly known as "Monkey Block." As landmarks that are no longer there go, this one was a doozy. Built in 1853, the Montgomery Block was for a time the largest and most prestigious commercial building on the West Coast, but it's not for commerce that it is remembered. A bar on the ground floor, called the Bank Exchange, gave the city its signature drink—pisco punch. Pisco is a Peruvian or Chilean brandy that perhaps was introduced locally by Chilean immigrants during the Gold Rush. To make pisco punch, pineapple was infused in gum syrup and mixed with water, lemon juice, and Pisco brandy to make an innocuous tasting beverage that packed something of a wallop. It was commonly observed that the drink could "make a gnat fight an elephant." The bar was done in by the Volstead Act in 1919, and the drink long ago fell out of favor. Of late, Pisco punch has begun reappearing on drink menus around town, thanks to today's inquisitive breed of bartenders. As the city grew, the Monkey Block's more status-conscious tenants moved down Montgomery St., and artists, tradesmen, musicians, writers, and poets moved in. By the 1880s, the immense building was the center of the city's bohemian life. In the basement was a public bath, habituated by writers such as the young Mark Twain, who worked as a reporter in town from 1864 until 1866. (Twain, having deserted the Confederate Army in 1861, spent much of the '60s in the West.) While bathing here Twain reputedly made the acquaintance of a fireman named Tom Sawyer and thought well enough of the name to use it in his best-known work. Ambrose Bierce, Jack London, and Robert Louis Stevenson all either worked in the building or had other excuses for dropping by. The building was demolished in 1959, and the site served as a parking lot for more than a decade before ground was broken for the Transamerica Pyramid.

● Turn left onto Montgomery. This first block has numerous landmark buildings, most obvious being the Old Transamerica Building (701 Montgomery St.), a flatiron clad in white terra-cotta tiles. It was built in 1911 for A. P. Giannini, founder of the Bank of Italy, which grew to become Bank of America. It's now the San Francisco headquarters for the Church of Scientology.

● Across the street, at 710 Montgomery, the Black Cat Cafe was a famous hangout for arty bohemians from 1933 until 1963. In the 1950s, drag-queen host(ess) José Sarria gained notoriety for his operatic performances here. A few doors down, at 716–720 Montgomery, Diego Rivera and Frida Kahlo lived and worked in fellow artist Ralph Stackpole's studios on and off throughout the 1930s. Stackpole's studios were the center of the city's artistic social scene since the early 1920s, and for a time photographer Dorothea Lange subleased a photography studio upstairs. The completely gutted building at 722

Hotaling Buildings with the Transamerica Pyramid in the background

49

Montgomery was the office of lawyer Melvin Belli from 1959 to 1989. Belli, himself a flamboyant character, represented clients such as Lenny Bruce and Zsa Zsa Gabor, as well as Jack Ruby for the murder of Lee Harvey Oswald. Belli helped broker the deal that brought the Rolling Stones to the Altamont Speedway in 1969, and scenes were shot in Belli's office for the film *Gimme Shelter*. He once appeared in an episode of *Star Trek,* in which he played a character named Gorgan. Belli was fond of pirates, or at least of certain swashbuckling traditions. He celebrated court victories by firing a canon from the roof of his building and he raised a Jolly Roger from a rooftop flagpole. He kept a human skeleton, which he called Elmer, in his office. He was married six times and lived a long life of 88 years (he died in 1996). The building was allowed to deteriorate after the 1989 earthquake, and its roof eventually caved in. In October 2009, the Belli family put it up for sale, priced at $10.5 million.

● Turn right at Jackson, and half a block down you'll reach the Hotaling Buildings (455 and 463–73 Jackson), which flank narrow Hotaling Place. Anson Parson Hotaling, who distributed liquor among other goods, built the stately offices at 455 Jackson, then bought the second building, which he used as a warehouse for his booze. When the buildings survived the 1906 quake and fire, a jaunty little rhyme was composed by one Charles K. Field:

> *If, as one says, God spanked the town*
> *For being overfrisky*
> *Why did He burn the churches down*
> *And save Hotaling's whisky?*

● The building at 415–31 Jackson St. was built in 1853 and once was home to Domingo Ghirardelli's chocolate company. In 1860, Ghirardelli added the structure at 407 Jackson. The older building, you'll notice, has some intriguing details, with faces watching out from the frames of the upstairs windows. The much plainer 1860 building seems to suggest Ghirardelli had his mind more on the bottom line as his business expanded.

● At Sansome St. turn left and then cut back up Gold St. Considering San Francisco owed its good fortune to the Gold Rush, it's interesting that Gold St. should turn out to be so inconspicuous. It's a narrow lane, one block long, much of it walled in by the back sides of brick buildings. One entrance leads to Bix, a spectacularly swank supper club that recreates the decadence and grandeur not of the Barbary Coast, but of the Jazz Age.

Turn right on Montgomery, then left onto Pacific St. It's an agreeable enough street to look at, with its perfectly silent historic buildings, but there's little to suggest how terrific the 400 and 500 blocks were more than a century ago. However, saunter up the 500 block for a peek into the entry of No. 555, graced by some lovely nudes embossed in plaster. Think of this detail as an overt tribute to the neighborhood's bawdy past. The building was once the location of the Hippodrome, a dance hall. The Hippodrome was across the street during its heyday, and moved to this location in time for World War II, when the district enjoyed a minor revival, thanks to the influx of military personnel embarking from the city.

At the junction of Pacific, Kearny, and Columbus, look across Columbus and you'll spot the Comstock Saloon, a lovely old establishment with a questionable past. It opened in 1907 as the Andromeda.

Head up Kearny toward Broadway. These are the declining remnants of modern sleazeville, with Kearny a lusterless adjunct of the Broadway strip-tease strip. You'll notice the Lusty Lady, a rare worker-owned strip joint. In the 1990s, the strippers here unionized and went on strike, and in 2003 they bought their bosses out. Apart from that, the place has an old-fashioned peep-show quality, with women behind glass putting on private shows for paying customers, who slide dollars into a slot to keep the show going.

At Broadway turn left. From the signs above the shops here, it is obvious that this is a very sex-minded street. Broadway looks great at night, when the neon creates a reassuring tent of light that obliterates the darkness overhead. At the corner of Broadway and Columbus, the Condor Club is once again a strip joint, after dallying in the food industry for the past two decades. In the 1960s it was the Taj Mahal of San Francisco's burlesque scene. Carol Doda's topless and bottomless act set the pace here. A plaque on the Columbus St. side of the building makes hay out of two landmark dates: June 16, 1964, when Ms. Doda first unveiled her ample bosom (which, with silicone enhancement, reputedly reached size 44D); and September 3, 1969, when she first shimmied out of her skivvies on stage. Fondly remembered by old-time San Franciscans is the Condor's sign, which featured a larger-than-life caricature of Doda with blinking red light bulbs for nipples. The Condor was the site of a grisly death, of the sort that makes people try not to snicker. One night after hours, in November 1983, a dancer and bouncer played hide the salami on top of a piano. The piano was supported by a hydraulic pole used to make it rise and fall during performances. One thing leading to another, as you might expect, the hydraulics were activated and the love-makers were crushed between the piano and the ceiling. The dancer survived. The bouncer didn't.

POINTS OF INTEREST

Bix 56 Gold St., 415-433-6300

Comstock Saloon 155 Columbus Ave., 415-617-0071

Lusty Lady 1033 Kearny St., 415-391-3991

Condor Club 560 Broadway, 415-781-8222

route summary

1. Start at Portsmouth Square, corner of Kearny and Washington streets.
2. Head down Washington, to the intersection of Montgomery St. and Columbus Ave.
3. Turn left on Montgomery St.
4. Turn right on Jackson St.
5. Turn left on Sansome St.
6. Turn left on Gold St.
7. Turn right on Montgomery St.
8. Turn left on Pacific Ave.
9. At the intersection of Kearny St. and Columbus Ave., cross Columbus.
10. Return to corner of Kearny St. and Pacific Ave., and head up Kearny, toward Broadway.
11. Turn left on Broadway.
12. End at the corner of Broadway and Columbus Ave.

The old Transamerica Building

Coit Tower

Greenwich St

Filbert St

Filbert St

Powell St

Jasper Pl

Genoa Pl

Varennes St

Sonoma St

Grant Ave

Alta St

Castle St

Montgomery St

Sansome St

finish

Washington Square Park

Union St

Union St

Green St

Green St

Green St

Kearny St

Vallejo St

Vallejo St

Bartol St

Vallejo St

Columbus Ave

Romolo Pl

Broadway

Osgood Pl

Mason St

Vallejo St

Powell St

Broadway

Pacific Ave

Stockton St

Pacific Ave

Grant Ave

Columbus Ave

Gold St

Trenton St

Jackson St

Jackson St

Wentworth Pl

John St

start

Washington St

Merchant St

0   100   200   300 yards

0   100   200   300 meters

7 NORTH BEACH: BOPPIN' DOWN THE BEAT PATH

BOUNDARIES: **Washington St., Powell St., Filbert St., Grant Ave.**
DISTANCE: **1 mile**
DIFFICULTY: **Easy**
PARKING: **There is an underground lot beneath Portsmouth Square, at Washington and Kearny streets, one block from the starting point.**
PUBLIC TRANSIT: **1, 10, 30X, 41 Muni buses**

North Beach no longer swarms with the goatee-and-beret crowd, and the Italian language is less commonly heard in the neighborhood than it once was. And yet the neighborhood continues to benefit from its heritage as an enclave of Beatniks and Italian immigrants. The chief links to the past are cafes and historic bars, which retain a somewhat earthy, European charm that no doubt appealed to the poets and painters of the Eisenhower years. Italian-American families still own most of the businesses, many of them after several generations. The off-kilter, diagonal slice of Columbus Ave., the main drag, and the closeness of Russian and Telegraph Hills, which rise above North Beach, make this quarter feel more intimate and self-contained than other parts of San Francisco. It's somewhat touristy, especially on weekends. Drop in on a weekday afternoon, or in time for lunch, and you'll get a more local sense of the area. Return at night and take the North Beach Barhopping Tour.

● Start at the foot of Columbus Ave., where the Financial District abruptly ends and North Beach gradually cranks up. Columbus Ave. mainlines into the neighborhood. The first sign of North Beach character is Caffè Macaroni, a cramped little Neapolitan trattoria at No. 59, where the waiters are notorious for flattering women who walk by. It's a bit early in the walk to stop and eat, but at least have a look at the menu and make a note to drop by for dinner sometime. This is a great local eatery.

● On the next block, on the opposite side of the street, the basement-level Purple Onion has been a neighborhood mainstay since 1952. Legendary comedy and folk music acts have taken its stage. Phyllis Diller and the Kingston Trio got their starts here. Jim Nabors sang in the club in his pre-Gomer days, and the owner, Bud Steinhoff, was in the habit of smashing glass when Nabors reached for high notes.

In the 1970s, Robin Williams worked the stage for tips. These days the Onion bills itself as a piano bar, but it still hosts comedy events.

● On the triangle formed by intersecting Columbus and Kearny stands the green copper-clad Columbus Tower, headquarters for Francis Ford Coppola's filmmaking company Zoetrope. Coppola bought the building in 1972, the year his film *The Godfather* was released. Coppola was already a fixture in the neighborhood, frequenting local bars and cafes. He keeps an office on the top floor, beneath the building's graceful cupola. (Incidentally, a *coppola,* in Italian, is a type of cap once popular amongst the common folk of Sicily.) Cafe Zoetrope, on the ground floor, is a fine spot for a pizza and a bottle of wine. Columbus Tower, originally called the Sentinel Building, was built for corrupt political boss Abe Reuf just after the '06 quake.

● A block up, Jack Kerouac Alley is named for the author of *On the Road* and other tomes of bop prose that captured the restlessness of the Beat Generation. It's a perfect alley for Kerouac, who liked to drink at Vesuvio, the bar that overlooks the alley. He also associated with poet Lawrence Ferlinghetti, whose City Lights bookstore is just across the alley. Ferlinghetti opened the shop in 1953. He made headlines in 1956 when he published a pocket edition of Allen Ginsberg's *Howl* and the poem was banned for containing obscenities. Ferlinghetti won a high-profile court battle and the book was put back on the shelves. City Lights is a great bookstore, so step inside and head upstairs to the intimate Poetry Room, where volumes of verse—Beat or otherwise—fill the shelves. Ferlinghetti's office is just off this little reading room, so you might even run into him.

● At Broadway, on the northwest corner, take a look at the *Jazz* mural, by Bill Weber and Tony Klaas. Clarinetist Benny Goodman (who was not a local figure) presides over a group of San Francisco characters, including Emperor Norton, Herb Caen, and some Italian fishermen.

● Turn right on Broadway. A block down, on the north side, step into the Beat Museum to look at Beat memorabilia and a collection of old editions by Kerouac, Ginsberg, Burroughs, and other Holy Goofs. Admission is $5. In the gift shop you can grab hip T-shirts and buttons declaring your Beatitude.

- Head left, up narrow Romolo Place for a look at North Beach's back-alley side, and turn left on Vallejo St. At Grant, make a caffeine stop at Caffè Trieste, a historic coffeehouse that has been run by Gianni Giotta since 1956. Giotta once aspired to sing opera, and he and his family still sing cantos in the small cafe on Saturday afternoons (call ahead to see if Papa Gianni is performing). Trieste has a comfortable, timeworn feel to it, and literary types have always dropped in to kickstart their muses. Francis Ford Coppola worked on his *Godfather* screenplay at one of the tables. The walls are covered with old photos. It's part family album, part celebrity schmoozefest—well worth studying over a cappuccino.

- Half a block up, at Vallejo and Columbus streets, the church of St. Francis of Assisi was built in 1860. It's the second-oldest Catholic church in the city, after Mission Dolores. Kitty-corner from the church, at 373 Columbus St., Molinari Delicatessen is a classic deli with hanging salamis, shelves of olives and table wines, and the tantalizing scent of dry cheese. Drop in for a whiff or to grab a sandwich, if you have visions of a picnic at the park later on. (This tour ends at a park.)

- Follow Columbus to Green St. and turn left. At No. 649, the Green Street Mortuary is notable for providing a marching band that leads funeral corteges through Chinatown. The marching band, led by Lisa Pollard, a.k.a. the "Saxlady," includes many local jazz musicians and even some members of the San Francisco Symphony. If they happen to be marching out as you pass by, quit this tour and follow the band, man.

- Across the street, take note of Club Fugazi, the attractive theater at No. 678. The zany send-up stage

Columbus Tower

productions of *Beach Blanket Babylon* have ruled the stage here since 1975. Years before that, the Beats put on poetry readings in the club. Next door, Capp's Corner is a friendly old neighborhood eatery that manages to hang on, despite changing tastes.

● Turn right on Powell St. and right again on Union St. Cross Columbus and turn right. This block is one of the street's busiest, alive with cafes and restaurants, including Caffè Roma, where the beans are roasted on the premises, and Rose Pistola, where contemporary Italian cuisine is served amid stylish, jazzy decor. No gut-busting portions here.

● Turn left on Green St. Halfway up the block, on the left side, is Caffè BaoNecci, a family-run establishment that typifies the way in which North Beach retains its intimate, old-world feel. The original owners, Danilo and Danila DiPiramo retired, and rather than close the shop they sold it to another couple, Walter and Stefania Gambaccini, in 2005. The place is still known to neighborhood old timers as Danilo Bakery, despite the name change. The Gambaccinis, from Altopascio, Italy, have broadened the menu to include panini, pizza, and pasta, which still relies heavily on the bakery's century-old oven. You can order a coffee and watch as neighbors drop by for fresh loaves.

● Turn left on Grant Ave., which plays second fiddle to Columbus Ave. but does so with a grace that should be instantly apparent. The narrow street is packed with shop fronts of all varieties, including clothing boutiques, antique dealers, grocers, restaurants, cafes, and bars. Study the window displays as you walk by and duck in wherever your curiosity is piqued. Be sure to make it all the way up to Aria, between Union and Filbert. It's a chaotic and densely packed antique store cut from the old curiosity shop cloth. The owner leads a charmed life, spending his time traveling the globe in search of interesting things to sell in his shop. There's no telling what you might find on any given visit, but the stock tends to range the realm of the unusual and unexpected.

● At Filbert turn left and walk down toward Washington Square. On the corner of Stockton, poke your head into Liguria, an admirably nondescript shop that sells just one thing: focaccia. In the age of one-stop shopping, this place constitutes the ultimate anachronism, but it manages to get by on the strength of a quality product. If you've been assembling the fixings for a picnic along this tour, be sure to add a warm half-sheet to your sack of victuals.

● Also overlooking the park is the church of Saints Peter and Paul. Crazily, the church's address is 666 Filbert St. It was built in 1924 and is very popular for weddings. Poet Ferlinghetti dubbed it the "marzipan church," and indeed its façade does have a cake-like aspect. Joe DiMaggio and Marilyn Monroe, unable to wed in the church due to an earlier Monroe divorce, snapped their wedding photos on the front steps after getting officially hitched at City Hall.

Washington Square itself is an odd-shaped square, as diagonal Columbus Ave. slices off a chunk of it, leaving a small triangular remainder on the west side of the street. Still, Washington Square is a nice patch of green with some trees and statues. Most interesting is the statue of Benjamin Franklin, erected in 1897 by a dentist named Henry D. Cogswell. Cogswell, an ardent prohibitionist, wasn't so much intent on honoring Franklin as he was on luring the town's heavy drinkers away from the bottle. Around the statue's base are water taps, with labels indicating the waters' sources—one indicates the water is from Vichy, France. The spouts have been out of order for decades now. Also in the square is a firemen's statue, put here by fire chaser Lillie Hitchcock Coit. (See the Telegraph Hill walk for more on her.) Pick a bench or a spot on the grass and settle in for a while. Your dogs must be tired.

POINTS OF INTEREST

Caffè Macaroni **59 Columbus Ave., 415-956-9737**

Purple Onion **140 Columbus Ave., 415-956-1610**

Cafe Zoetrope **916 Kearny St., 415-291-1700**

City Lights Books **261 Columbus Ave., 415-362-8193**

Beat Museum **540 Broadway, 415-399-9626**

Caffè Trieste **601 Vallejo St., 415-392-6739**

Molinari Delicatessen **373 Columbus Ave., 415-421-2337**

Capp's Corner **1600 Powell St., 415-989-2589**

Rose Pistola **532 Columbus Ave., 415-399-0499**

Caffè BaoNecci **516 Green St., 415-989-1806**

Aria **1522 Grant Ave., 415-433-0219**

Liguria **1700 Stockton St., 415-421-3786**

Sts. Peter and Paul Church **666 Filbert St., 415-421-0809**

route summary

1. Begin at the southern end of Columbus and head north, into the neighborhood.
2. Turn right at Broadway.
3. Head up Romolo Place.
4. Turn left at Vallejo St.
5. Turn right at Columbus Ave.
6. Turn left at Green St.
7. Turn right at Powell St.
8. Turn right at Union St.
9. Turn right at Columbus Ave.
10. Turn left at Green St.
11. Turn left at Grant St.
12. Turn left at Filbert St.
13. Walk to Washington Square, corner of Stockton and Filbert streets.

Vesuvio's self-deprecating sign

Filbert St

Washington
Square Park

Stockton St

Union St

start

Columbus Ave

Powell St

Green St

Jasper Pl

Bannam Pl

Grant Ave

Varennes St

Sonoma St

Kearny St

Union St

Castle St

Montgomery St

Green St

Kearny St

Margrave Pl
Grant Ave

Vallejo St

Fresno St

Vallejo St

Stockton St

Columbus Ave

Romolo Pl

Broadway

Broadway

Jack
Kerouac
Alley

finish

Pacific Ave

Powell St

Cordelia St

Pacific Ave

Beckett St

Columbus Ave

Jackson St

0   50   100   150 yards
0   50   100   150 meters

8 NORTH BEACH BARS: IN SEARCH OF THE 90-PROOF MUSE

BOUNDARIES: **Union St, Columbus Ave, Grant Ave, Jack Kerouac Alley**
DISTANCE: **Approx. ¾ mile**
DIFFICULTY: **Easy (and getting easier)**
PARKING: **Driving is not a good idea if you're drinking, but there is a parking lot on Vallejo between Columbus and Mason.**
PUBLIC TRANSIT: **The 30 and 41 Muni buses pass through North Beach.**

North Beach is one of San Francisco's best neighborhoods for barhopping, simply because the district contains a variety of fine watering holes within a small, walkable area. The offerings range from rowdy local taverns to historic beatnik dives, and the crowds tend to be a diverse mix of city slickers, sozzled poets, and chatty tourists. While it would be irresponsible to drink in every bar on this tour, your throat is liable to be a bit dry at some point during your walk and you'll want stop and have one here or there. If on occasion you choose to do the lawyerly thing—passing the bar instead of drinking in it—have a vicarious libation and be sure to return for the real thing another time. The best time to hit the bars in North Beach is the latter half of the week, when things are on the upswing, but not on the weekend, when the bridge-and-tunnel crowd invades the neighborhood. Late afternoon or early evening can be quite nice, if you're inclined toward enjoying a drink or two before a meal.

● **Mario's Bohemian Cigar Store**, on the corner of Columbus Ave. and Union St., is always a good place to start for its central location and its early hours. Mario's is a friendly joint with a limited menu, so you can get some carbohydrates under your belt here. The toasted focaccia sandwiches are excellent. It gets its name from the late Mario Crismani, a retired cop from Trieste, Italy, who opened the place in 1972. You'll spot photos of him and his family above the bar. Signore Mario also served as president of the city's Bocce Ball Association. The bar once really did sell cigars, and it was originally a hangout for older Italian gents. These days, the crowd is younger and more mixed, and of course there is no smoking. Other than that, the place hasn't changed a bit.

● After departing Mario's, saunter east on down Union St. to Stockton St. and turn right. Midway up the block is a classy little joint called Tony Nik's. If you didn't know any better, you'd think this spot was a smart little retro knock-off, inspired by *Goodfellas* or some other mobster movie. Most of the joint's current regulars were born after Frank traded in his brown toupee for a silver one. But Tony Nik's ain't no knock off. The decor is of genuine Rat Pack vintage. The best time to come is for Happy Hour (4–7 p.m.).

● At Green St., hook left and in less than a block you'll reach Gino and Carlo, one of North Beach's enduring neighborhood bars. This place is purely local, in the best possible way. It's nothing fancy but always lively and newcomers will feel welcome. It has some history, too. Long ago, hard-drinking *Chronicle* columnist Charles McCabe—known as the "Fearless Spectator"—regularly penned his daily column from a table here. And rock singer Janis Joplin reputedly frequented the bar in the '60s. The drinks are relatively cheap, there's a pool table and pinball machine, and usually there's a game on T.V.

● At Grant Ave., turn right and head for the Saloon, just past Vallejo St. It's the oldest bar in San Francisco, having opened its doors in 1861. Originally called Wagner's Beer Hall, it is a true survivor—it has endured the demise of the Barbary Coast, the '06 quake, the Prohibition era, and the 1960s. Most of the tosspots who patronize the place are survivors of one kind or another as well. The Saloon, bless it, is no model of gentrification. It's dusty, sagging, and peeling. The faded painted ladies over the bar lack Victorian propriety. But the overall vibe is good. At night, the Saloon features live blues bands—good ones, usually.

● Head up narrow Fresno St. and then right on Romolo Place. 15 Romolo is the address and the name of a sultry little hideaway that opened in the late 1990s. Before that, the place was a Basque restaurant. It's a contemporary watering hole without pretense. The barkeeps are keeping up with the current renaissance in mixology, and the drink list regularly introduces original concoctions and "seasonal" cocktails along with updated classics.

● Romolo Place leads to Broadway, with its garish neon signs and strip-show barkers. You'll notice they don't make barkers like they used to. These guys and dolls seem listless, and don't bark much. Enrico's, just half a block to the left, is a North Beach institution that opened in 1959. If you're just drinking go inside and head for the bar. There's usually a singer or jazz combo performing. Dining here is a fairly costly proposition, and the food gets mixed reviews, but if you're strolling by around lunchtime, drop into the adjacent lunch counter, Naked Lunch, for soup and a sandwich, which you can enjoy on Enrico's beloved sidewalk patio.

● Backtrack to Columbus. Hopefully you've still got your sea legs beneath you, because we're following the fireworks show model and have saved the biggest splash for last. Turn left, and left again on the squib of a street called William Saroyan Place (named after the author). If you can't find Specs', friend, you're finished. Hopefully that's not the case. Specs' is a little grotto that oozes atmosphere without trying much. Someone took the trouble to outfit the place with curios from every port of the South Seas, but that was decades ago. The place is a dark and dusty museum of the best possible sort, filled with the lurid and the arcane. The crowd is a jovial mix of juiced philosophers and loosened-tie types.

● Just beyond William Saroyan Place is Tosca. Like any great bar or church, Tosca has been around forever and attracts a healthy cross-section of society. The place has a slightly aloof dignity. A sepia hue lingers over the ceiling from decades of cigarette smoke, the old jukebox plays only Italian arias, and the red leatherette booths show very little wear despite their obvious mid-20th-century vintage. Bob Dylan and Alan Ginsberg were thrown out of the bar in 1965 after a companion walked into the ladies' room, but these days Tosca is far more accommodating to its celebrity patrons. Sean Penn and Francis Ford Coppola often entertain in the clubby back room.

● On the opposite side of Columbus Ave., two Beat landmarks, Vesuvio and City Lights Bookstore, flank narrow Jack Kerouac Alley. They don't serve drinks at City Lights, so bop on over to Vesuvio. It's a beauty of a bar that somewhat resembles a Galway pub, though surely that was never intended. The place has its own native eccentricity and a place in North Beach history. It opened in 1949, and when in town, writers such as Kerouac and poet Dylan Thomas drank and told fish tales here. Owner Henri Lenoir traded in on the Beatnik craze by marketing a kit that included a beret and a false goatee. The place still has the spirit. Sit downstairs to soak in the bar's history or at an upstairs window to watch Columbus Ave. flow by.

POINTS OF INTEREST

Mario's Bohemian Cigar Store **566 Columbus Ave., 415-362-0536**

Tony Nik's **1534 Stockton St., 415-693-0993**

Gino and Carlo **548 Green St., 415-421-0896**

Saloon **1232 Grant Ave., 415-989-7666**

15 Romolo **15 Romolo Place, 415-398-1359**

Enrico's **504 Broadway, 415-982-6223**

Naked Lunch **504 Broadway, 415-577-4951**

Specs' **12 William Saroyan Place, 415-421-4112**

Tosca Cafe **242 Columbus Ave., 415-391-1244**

Vesuvio **255 Columbus Ave., 415-362-3370**

ROUTE SUMMARY

1. Begin at Mario's, corner of Union St. and Columbus Ave.
2. Head up Union St. to Stockton St. and turn right to reach Tony Nik's.
3. Turn left at Green St. to reach Gino and Carlo's.
4. Turn right at Grant Ave. to reach the Saloon.
5. Turn left at Fresno St.
6. Turn right at Romolo Place to reach 15 Romolo Place.
7. Turn left at Broadway to reach Enrico's.
8. Backtrack on Broadway to Columbus Ave. and turn left.
9. Turn into William Saroyan Place for Specs'.
10. Stay on Columbus Ave. for Tosca.
11. Cross Columbus Ave. and walk to Jack Kerouac Alley to reach Vesuvio.

The Saloon

Pfeiffer St

Chestnut St

Fielding St

Grant Ave

Lombard St

Lombard St

Lombard St

Pioneer Park

Greenwich Steps

Greenwich St

Battery St

Stockton St

Child St

Edith St

Greenwich St

Coit Tower

Filbert St

Powell St

Filbert St

start

Filbert St

Alta St

Calhoun Ter

Sansome St

Icehouse Aly

Washington Square Park

Genoa Pl

Kearny St

Castle St

Filbert St

Union St

Varennes St

Sonoma St

Union St

Columbus Ave

Jasper Pl

Grant Ave

Bannam Pl

Green St

Green St

Montgomery St

Bartol St

Vallejo St

Powell St

finish

Vallejo St

Stockton St

Vallejo St

Fresno St

Kearny St

Columbus Ave

Broadway

Pacific Ave

0   100   200   300 yards

0   100   200   300 meters

9 TeLeGraPH HILL: SCaLInG THe STairWays TO ParaDISe

BOUNDARIES: **Stockton St., Greenwich St., Sansome St., Vallejo St.**
DISTANCE: **1½ miles**
DIFFICULTY: **Strenuous**
PARKING: **Off-street parking is available on Vallejo St., between Stockton and Powell streets, opposite the police station. Curbside parking is very difficult to find and limited to two hours Monday through Saturday.**
PUBLIC TRANSIT: **30, 41, 45 Muni buses**

On most days Telegraph Hill feels like San Francisco's Shangri-La with its wooden stairways zigzagging up hills too steep for paved streets. Walkers are naturally drawn to the steps, which weave through dense gardens and past Victorian houses both humble and refined. This little refuge tells us the rest of San Francisco hasn't taken full advantage of its spectacularly impractical topography. Telegraph Hill wasn't always so pretty a spot, however. Its east face was once a rock quarry overlooking a fleet of rotting ships. By the early 20th century, the hillside had become a de facto dumping ground. Beginning in the 1950s, the hill's bohemian inhabitants transformed their hidden quarter, mostly through tasteful and imaginative landscaping. The neighborhood is fairly hoity now, thanks to escalating real estate values, but it continues to offer the city's best walking. A good time to walk this one is on a lightly overcast morning, when details are drawn out from the shadows beneath the trees.

● The hill slopes up from North Beach, so we'll start at Washington Square, on the corner of Filbert and Stockton, and walk a block over to Greenwich. Just before you reach Greenwich, the arts and crafts Swiss chalet at 1736 Stockton is the Maybeck Building. Berkeley-based Bernard Maybeck, one of California's most influential architects, designed the building in 1907. It was originally the Telegraph Hill Neighborhood House, which offered services to immigrant families. Enter into a shady courtyard, which is a pleasant composition with a brick patio surrounded by varying inner faces of the building.

● At Greenwich St., turn right and head up (and up and up). At Grant, turn right and half a block down, at Gerte Alley, you'll get an attractive preview of Coit Tower. It's a more than adequate excuse for breaking up the upward trek. Back on Greenwich head up the steps through Pimentell Garden, named for Samantha Pimentell who tended the flora here for 25 years. The steps lead to Telegraph Hill Blvd., on which cars spiral up to the summit. Rather than follow the road, look on the other side for the stone steps that lead to the top.

● Pioneer Park, on the leveled summit of Telegraph Hill, is where you'll find Coit Tower and a statue of Christopher Columbus, which was a gift from Columbus' hometown of Genoa, Italy. The explorer, who for better or worse got so many things rolling in the Americas, never laid eyes on San Francisco Bay, but this bronze likeness appears to be admiring the view of it. You ought to do the same. The vantage here is as wide as it gets, ranging from the Golden Gate to the west and on past Treasure Island to the east. In the early days of San Francisco, the arrival of ships entering the Golden Gate was observed from this lookout, and through semaphore signals the news, along with the type of ship, was "telegraphed" (thus the hill's name) to the bustling downtown clustered on

Back Story: Wild Parrots

The parrots you're likely to see on Telegraph Hill are cherry-head conures, which first appeared here in the late 1970s or early 1980s. Many were either released or escaped from captivity, but a sizeable portion were born wild in San Francisco. Mark Bittner, author of *The Wild Parrots of Telegraph Hill* and subject of the documentary film of the same name, squatted in a former artist's shack on Greenwich St. for many years, studying and getting to know the birds. The book and film are highly recommended for anyone desiring a fascinating perspective on Telegraph Hill.

Yerba Buena Cove. Touts would sail or row out to meet the ships as they slowly proceeded into the bay. The city's economy revolved around shipping, and the bulk of the population would rush to the docks to greet each ship as it tied in.

- Coit Tower is visible from just about anywhere to the east of Nob and Russian hills, and is one of the city's more puzzling architectural monuments. A fluted column topped by an arched observatory, it was originally derided by locals, who saw it as a sore thumb. San Franciscans are notoriously negative when it comes to new structures invading their skyline, but the city eventually came around to accepting this one. It looks particularly attractive at night, when it's illuminated by lamps beaming up from the ground. It bears the name of Lillie Hitchcock Coit, who funded the project through an endowment specified in her will. Coit (1843–1929) was raised in San Francisco and became a big fan of a company of volunteer firefighters called Knickerbocker Engine Company No. 5. In those days, multiple companies would respond to fire alarms, and it was a competition to see which company arrived at a scene first to put out the fire. Some citizens, such as young Lillie, cheered on their favorite companies much as sports fans cheer on their favorite teams. Coit's passion for Knickerbocker No. 5 far surpassed the norm, however, and by the age of 20 she had become an honorary member of the company. She considered it a point of honor to appear at every fire along with her beloved crew of smoke-eaters. Consequently, many have speculated that Coit Tower was designed to resemble a firehose nozzle, but architect Henry T. Howard always maintained this was not his intention.

- You can enter Coit Tower free of charge and circle the lobby to inspect the beautiful WPA murals, which were added a year after the tower's completion in 1933. These frescoes sparked a huge controversy, as many of them have Socialist undertones. Some of the scenes depict laborers struggling to keep up with the demands of industry. Some of the more overt details in the original works were censored before the murals were unveiled.

- Exit the tower, descend the front steps, turn right, and look for the street sign for Greenwich St. This leads not to a paved road, but to some brick steps. Follow these down through dense greenery all the way to Montgomery St. Turn left at the bottom of the stairs and you'll reach Julius' Castle, one of the hill's kookier structures. This turreted fortress was the dreamchild of restaurateur Julius Roz, who opened the establishment in 1922. It closed in 2009, after operating for nearly nine decades.

● From the castle, walk along the east side of Montgomery past two buildings and find steps cutting back and then down Greenwich St., a pretty darn peaceful hideaway. These gardens here are the main attraction for the neighborhood's flock of parrots, who you'll often hear squawking in the canopy overhead. At 231 Greenwich you'll see some wooden steps to the right. Head up a little ways for an up-close look at some rusticated shacks that reflect the old neighborhood's bohemian past, and then return to the Greenwich Steps and head down to the bottom. At Sansome St., turn right and walk one block to Filbert St.

● From the bottom of Filbert it should be instantly obvious that you have your work cut out for you. A concrete and metal stairway ascends a sheer cliff carved out by rock quarrying in the 19th century. Flowers cling to the cliffside, thanks to adventurous gardeners who rappelled down to plant seedlings.

● From the top of the cliff rustic wooden steps lead into the Grace Marchant Gardens, which are the most elaborate and lovingly tended gardens on the hill. Grace Marchant, a retired Hollywood stuntwoman, resided at the corner of Filbert and Napier Lane, where in 1950 she began the gardens that now flourish here. Her daughter, Valletta, took on a similar mission on Greenwich St. Today, the gardens are tended by neighborhood volunteers. The land itself belongs to the city.

● A wood plank walkway leads down narrow Napier Lane, where we ought to make a short detour, for this is surely the sweetest cul de sac in all San Francisco. Little more than a footpath, it accesses a row of small houses shaded by trees. Farther up Filbert, Darrell Place is a similarly narrow, though paved, lane.

● At the top of the block, the Art Deco apartment building at 1360 Montgomery appeared in the 1947 film *Dark Passage*, starring Humphrey Bogart and Lauren Bacall. The building stood in for Bacall's apartment, where she allowed the fugitive Bogart to hide out. Scenes in the neighborhood reveal that the steps weren't nearly so beautiful then as they are today. The silver nautical motifs on the building's side make it instantly recognizable and also make it a good photo op. The film is well worth watching.

Back Story:
In the Kitchen with Dyna

For many years rock was blasted out of Telegraph Hill's eastern side by a company called Gray Brothers. Using dynamite, the company regularly shook the foundations of the workingmen's cottages above, and in some instances the blasts actually destroyed homes. Property on the hill, though very central, was affordable to dock hands because the grades were too steep to attract the wealthy. The Gray Brothers intended to continue quarrying until Telegraph Hill was completely flattened, along the way buying out neighbors upset by the disturbance of daily blasts. Once the hill was flattened, real estate values would naturally increase, and the Gray Brothers could then sell the land for top dollar. Telegraph Hill residents fought back, getting a court injunction to stop the blasting, and when Gray Brothers defied the court, the neighbors rolled rocks down on the company, to slow their progress. Eventually, one of the Gray Brothers was killed by an employee of the company, putting a stop to rock quarrying on Telegraph Hill.

- Turn left onto Montgomery and left again half a block later, onto historic Alta St. On the south side of the block, the red-brick house with upstairs galleries at 31 Alta was a speakeasy during Prohibition. On the north side, the house at 60–64 Alta is known as the Duck House, for the ducks painted beneath the eaves. Author Armistead Maupin lived in one of the building's apartments in the early 1970s, and actor Rock Hudson reputedly visited him here.

- Alta dead-ends, so backtrack to Montgomery, turn left, and turn left again onto Union St., which leads to a nub called Calhoun Terrace. Here some of the city's oldest houses rub shoulders with modern masterpieces. The Kahn House, at 66 Calhoun, is the work of Richard Neutra, the architect often credited with introducing the International Style of modern architecture to California. His cliffhanger doesn't look at all out of place here, and its expansive windows fully exploit the view of the bay. For the best vantage point, walk a little ways down the Union St. steps and look up at Neutra's building. Loop around to the upper side of Calhoun. The house at 9 Calhoun was built in 1854—very early days for this city—and it has been lovingly restored.

● Return to Montgomery St. and meander back down to North Beach. Half a block past Union, Montgomery dead-ends and the steps leading down afford a perfect perspective of the Transamerica Pyramid and the Financial District skyline. Turn right onto Green St. and left onto Kearny St. For the heck of it, cut down San Antonio Place, which has no sign and looks like an entry to an apartment building's parking garage. It loops through the buildings, opening onto the Vallejo St. steps. Turn right and it's a straight shot to Caffè Trieste, where an espresso or beer surely has your name on it.

POINTS OF INTEREST

Coit Tower 1 Telegraph Hill Blvd., 415-362-0808

Julius' Castle 1541 Montgomery St, 415-392-2222

Caffè Trieste 601 Vallejo St, 415-392-6739

route summary

1. Start at the corner of Stockton and Filbert streets.

2. Walk one block north on Stockton St.

3. Turn right at Greenwich St.

4. At Grant turn right and walk half a block to Gerte St., then return to Greenwich St.

5. Walk up to Coit Tower and Pioneer Park.

6. Look for the sign to Greenwich St., at the top of Greenwich Steps, and walk down the steps.

7. At Montgomery St., along the east side of the street, look for the continuation of the Greenwich Steps.

8. At Sansome St. turn right.

9. At Filbert St. turn right and ascend the steps.

10. Take a quick detour onto Napier Lane.

11. At Montgomery St., turn left.

12. Take a detour onto Alta St. and then continue on Montgomery St.

13. Take a detour onto Union St. and Calhoun Terrace, then continue on Montgomery St.

14. Turn right onto Green St.

15. Turn left onto Kearny St.

16. Follow San Antonio Place, which leads to the Vallejo Steps.

17. Turn right onto Vallejo, following it down to the corner of Grant Ave.

Julius' Castle

Jackson St

Taylor St

Mason St

Jones St

Washington St

Washington St

Wetmore St

Codman Pl

Powell St

start

Clay St

Priest St

Clay St

Taylor St

Sproule Ln

Sacramento St

Pleasant St

Leroy Pl

Sacramento St

finish

Huntington Park

Cushman St

Jones St

California St

Mason St

Vine Ter

Nob Hill Cir

California St

0	50	100	150 yards
0	50	100	150 meters

Pine St

10 NOB HILL: HIGH ALTITUDE HIGH JINX

BOUNDARIES: **Washington St., Mason St., California St., Jones St.**
DISTANCE: **Approx. ¾ mile**
DIFFICULTY: **Mildly strenuous**
PARKING: **St. Mary's garage, California St. and Grant Ave.**
PUBLIC TRANSIT: **Powell-Mason cable car**

The nabobs and their opulent mansions are long gone, but Nob Hill still has a prestigious air about it. In the 1870s, soon after the advent of cable cars simplified getting up the hill from downtown, the silver kings and railroad barons moved in. Three decades later, the 1906 quake turned their privileged perch into an ash heap. High-class hotels, a lovely park, and awe-inspiring Grace Cathedral now stand where San Francisco's robber barons once lived. Add to the mix a handful of unexpected curiosities and you've got yourself a dandy little tour.

- Since Nob Hill began with the development of cable cars, we'll start our tour at the Cable Car Museum, on the corner of Washington and Mason streets. If you're a perfectionist, you can take the Powell-Mason cable car and get off directly in front of the museum. This is more than a historic site—it's the powerhouse that makes all the cable cars move. Inside, take a look at the system of wheels that turns the cables like spindles in a cassette tape. These cables run under the tracks of the entire system. Each individual car moves by gripping onto a cable, which pulls it up or down a street. Exhibits here demonstrate how the system works and also include some historic cable cars and photos.

- Head up Mason St. for two blocks to reach the summit of Nob Hill. At the corner of Sacramento St. just about everything we've climbed these heights to inspect comes into view. At 1000 Mason St. are the stately Brocklebank Apartments, which were featured in the Hitchcock film *Vertigo*. James Stewart, waiting behind the wheel of his car, began stalking Kim Novak when she emerged from this building.

- Across the street, the imposing Fairmont Hotel is one of many eye-catching buildings on Nob Hill. It's on the site of silver king James Fair's mansion, which was torn down by Fair's daughter before the quake of '06. The hotel she built on the site was nearly completed when the quake and fire turned it into a burned-out hull. Architect Julia Morgan drew the plans to restore the hotel, which finally opened a year to the day after the quake. Enter the Fairmont's grand lobby, have a seat in a plush chair, pretend you're waiting for someone, and admire the marble columns and stately stairs. Then poke around a bit. Peer into the swank Venetian Room restaurant, study the charming dated murals of circus performers in the otherwise dowdy Cirque Bar (designed by Timothy Pflueger), and ride the glass elevator to the top of the Fairmont's tower for a spectacular view. For the hotel's biggest surprise, you'll have to head down to the basement. Here you'll find the Tonga Room, a tiki bar that spared no expense when it came to the decor. The walls are fake lava rock, thatched roofs cover the tables, drinks are served in plastic coconut shells, and every 30 minutes a simulated monsoon strikes. At this writing, the Tonga's fate is uncertain. The hotel's owners are entertaining notions of converting this wing into high-end condominiums, while local tiki aficionados have gathered behind the cause of saving it. If it's still here, time your visit for happy hour and order a mai tai.

● Back outside, keep your ears peeled for the sound of the California St. cable car. It's the oldest of the surviving lines, having begun service April 10, 1878.

● Continue on Mason to California St. At the southeast corner of the Mason and California intersection stands the Mark Hopkins Hotel. Mark Hopkins was among the Big Four railroad barons and his mansion—which photos reveal to have been the hill's most extravagant—stood on this site. The mansion was a quake casualty, but the stone retaining wall survives. Note the way this building and the Brocklebank Apartments a block away, complement one another. The main attraction at the Mark Hopkins is the Top of the Mark, a snazzy bar with 360-degree views, a martini menu that's several pages long, and jazz combos several nights a week.

● The distinguished brownstone mansion across the street from the Fairmont belonged to James Flood, the shrewd saloon keeper who made his fortune on the Comstock Lode. Walk along California St. to get a good look at it. The 1906 quake and fire failed to bring the mansion down, but significant restoration was required; Willis Polk designed the additions. The Pacific Union Club, one of the city's most exclusive, has owned the house since 1906.

● Make a left onto California St. Pleasant Huntington Park shares the block with the Flood Mansion. It's a good spot to claim a park bench and admire Grace Cathedral, across the street. The park's *Tortoise Fountain* and *Dancing Sprites* bronze sculptures are also worth looking at for half a minute or so.

● Rather than head directly to Grace Cathedral, cross California St. The Huntington Hotel, another of San Francisco's finest, stands on the southeast corner. From here, your eye may naturally drift over to the Masonic Memorial Temple, on the southwest corner. Don't fight that impulse. The building isn't exactly beautiful, but it is adorned by some impressive art, most notably the immense 45- by 48-foot "endomosaic" window in the lobby. Artist Emile Norman invented the style, pressing crushed glass, sea shells, soil, and other materials between sheets of translucent plastic. The art is illuminated from behind by sunlight, giving it the vibrancy of a projected Kodachrome slide. After two years of working on it, Norman completed his endomosaic in 1957. It depicts Masonic history in California with typically mysterious symbols and a starkly twisted 1950s style. During business hours you can enter for a close look.

● Now cross California St. and visit Grace Cathedral. Before entering, pause to inspect the bronze doors, which are lovely copies of Lorenzo Ghiberti's *Doors of Paradise* in Florence, Italy. Tuck in your shirt and go inside. (The cathedral requests a $5 donation.) The cathedral, lofty enough to stage a dogfight between two small bi-planes (though such a spectacle has yet to occur), was erected on the charred grounds of the mansion of Charles Crocker, a Big Four magnate. The cathedral was designed by Lewis P. Hobart, who studied at the École des Beaux Arts in Paris. It was built not of stone,

Grace Cathedral

but of formed concrete. Construction began not long after the '06 quake and was completed in 1964. While inside, direct your peepers to the elegant and awesome 25-foot-wide rose window, above the main entrance.

- From here, emerge onto Taylor St., return to Sacramento St., and turn left for a look at some relatively modest but still eye-pleasing residential architecture. The bougainvillea-clad apartments at 1230 and 1242 Sacramento have an elegant, Belle Époque Parisian style. On the corner of Jones, at 1298 Sacramento St., the Chambord Apartments are well loved for their extravagant rounded balconies that call to mind Gaudí's ebullient style.

- For contrast, finish this tour by following Jones St. down into the Tenderloin. Despite the so-called "Tender-Nob" transition zone, the change from highfalutin' hilltop to lowlife slum is pretty astonishing.

POINTS OF INTEREST

Cable Car Museum 1201 Mason St., 415-474-1887

Fairmont Hotel 950 Mason St., 415-772-5000

Tonga Room 950 Mason St., 415-772-5278

Mark Hopkins Hotel 999 California St., 415-392-3434

Top of the Mark 999 California St., 415-616-6916

Masonic Memorial Temple 1111 California St., 415-776-4702

Grace Cathedral 1100 California St., 415-749-6300

route summary

1. Start at the corner of Mason and Washington streets.
2. Walk up Mason St. to Sacramento St., to the top of Nob Hill.
3. Continue on Mason St. to California St.
4. Turn left on California St.
5. Walk through Huntington Park.
6. At the corner of Taylor and California streets, cross over to the Masonic Temple.
7. Re-cross California St. to Grace Cathedral.
8. Emerge onto Taylor St. and turn left.
9. Turn left on Sacramento St.
10. Turn left on Jones St. and follow it down.

Cable Car Museum and cable car

Francisco St

Columbus Ave

Chestnut St

Powell St

Chestnut St

Jones St

Mason St

Lombard St

Chestnut St

George
Sterling
Park

Lombard St

Taylor St

start

Greenwich St

Columbus Ave

Hyde St

Greenwich St

Valparaiso St

Leavenworth St

Filbert St

Filbert St

Filbert St

Union St

Havens St

August Aly

Hyde St

Union St

Mason St

Allen St

Macondray Ln

Taylor St

Green St

Eastman Pl

Russell St

Jones St

Vallejo St

finish

Green St

| 0 | 100 | 200 | 300 yards |
| 0 | 100 | 200 | 300 meters |

11 russian Hill: PONDering THe curvy Street DISPUTe ON HIDDeN HILLTOP Lanes

BOUNDARIES: **Hyde St., Lombard St., Mason St., Vallejo St.**
DISTANCE: **1¼ miles**
DIFFICULTY: **Strenuous (steep hills)**
PARKING: **Street parking is nearly impossible to find and is limited to two hours.**
PUBLIC TRANSIT: **The Hyde St. cable car stops at the starting point of this tour. The 41 and 45 Union buses stop at Hyde St. just a few blocks away.**

Russian Hill is more hilly than it is Russian—in fact, not one fur hat did we see while walking the streets of this part of town while researching this book. (The name supposedly comes from shadowy rumors of Russian sailors who were buried here ages ago.) This was once a bohemian enclave, and it retains much of its quirkiness—in large part due to the neighborhood's uncompromising topography. Russian Hill is not at all conducive to the grid system in which downtown San Francisco's streets are laid out, so some streets simply dead-end, giving way to narrow footpaths and stairwells. This did not stop San Franciscans from building their houses here, and today it seems the more inaccessible the house, the more desirable the property. Gardeners have made the most of the neighborhood's secluded pedestrian zones, and walkers are likely to marvel that such tranquility is to be found so near the dense heart of the city.

● **Begin at the top of the curvy block of Lombard St.—commonly billed, with sideshow hyperbole, as the "crookedest street in the world." Russian Hill's best known landmark is a tidy, picture-perfect example of urban landscaping. Gardeners tend to yawn at the choice of planting, which looks like the work of a fussy old granny. Meanwhile some locals argue that this isn't even the curviest street in the city. The other candidate, Vermont St. between McKinley and 22nd streets, at the foot of Potrero Hill, has five full turns and two half turns crammed into a single city block. Lombard has eight turns. Decision goes to Lombard. As you walk the curvy steps down, marvel over these facts: the hill has a 27-percent grade; the street originally ran straight down it; the curves were introduced in 1922 to slow down cars and to beautify the street; the postcards began to appear soon after that.**

● After negotiating that last curve, turn left onto Leavenworth St. and then right on Chestnut St. The San Francisco Art Institute beckons. It's architecturally interesting, exhibiting the hallmarks of Spanish revival, such as a tower and a courtyard, while being built almost entirely of formed concrete. But the real attraction here is the Diego Rivera Gallery, featuring a fresco by the master himself. Rivera painted it in 1931 and called it *The Making of a Fresco Showing a Building of a City*. You'll notice Rivera painted himself into the scene. The gallery can be reached by walking through the courtyard. The Institute's photography department, founded by Ansel Adams in 1945, was the first college program devoted to fine-art photography. Photographers Dorothea Lange, Imogen Cunningham, and Minor White all taught here. So did painters Clyfford Still and Robert Stackpole. Former students include painter Richard Diebenkorn, sculptor Sargeant Johnson, photographer Annie Leibovitz, graffiti artist Barry McGee, and musicians Jerry Garcia and Courtney Love.

● Continue down Chestnut St. to Columbus Ave., the Main Street of North Beach. From the corner, you'll spot the marquee of Bimbo's 365 Club, one of the swankiest live music clubs in San Francisco. It's famous for the girl, clad in her birthday suit, who swims for hours in a fishbowl. No one has ever sufficiently explained how she got in the fish bowl, or why she doesn't need to come up for air. Bimbo's has been operating on this spot since 1951 and retains much of its fun, swingin' vibe. In an earlier location, at 365 Market St., a young Rita Hayworth danced in the club's chorus line.

● From this corner follow Taylor St. uphill for several blocks. Stay on the right side of the street. After crossing Union St. be on the lookout for a wooden staircase heading skywards from the sidewalk. This is not a private entrance—it is Macondray Lane, an actual city street (you'll spot the street sign). Climb on up. Macondray inspired author Armistead Maupin's "Barbary Lane" in *Tales of the City*. Stroll the deeply shaded footpath—which switches from wood steps to rough-cut stone to brick—and you'll see why this is one of the least urban streets in the city. It's lined on one side with nondescript Victorian houses, and local gardeners have turned some of the terraced spaces here into jungles of bamboo, tree ferns, and ponds. Ina Coolbrith, a poet and literary socialite, hosted her legendary salon at 15 Macondray Lane during the early 20th century. Coolbrith later had a park named for her, which we'll visit on this tour.

Follow Macondray past Jones St. to Leavenworth and turn left. At Green St. turn left again. This is a historic block, with twelve buildings listed on the National Register. Nearly every house on the south side of the street predates the 1906 earthquake and fire. The obvious standout is number 1067, the Feusier Octagon House. Built in 1857–59, this was one of many eight-sided homes built in San Francisco (another can be seen on the Marina and Cow Hollow Walk). Orson S. Fowler, a phrenologist, developed the idea of octagon houses, saying they let in more light and offered improved ventilation. The mansard roof and dormers were added in the 1880s. The house at 1055 Green was built around 1866. It was originally an unassuming Italianate house, but in 1915 it was completely remodeled by Julia Morgan, who turned it into a Beaux Arts villa with stucco siding and a beautiful cast-iron balcony. Across the street, the charming Swiss Chalet at 1088 Green was originally a firehouse—Engine House No. 31. It was built in 1907.

Turn right at Jones St. Two ramps to your left link Jones to a short block of Vallejo St., adding to the secluded feel of this charmed cul-de-sac. The ramps, designed by Willis Polk in 1914, were commissioned not by the city but by a wealthy resident of the block. Polk also designed the lovely shingle-sided Craftsman house at 1015–19 Vallejo St. For a good vantage of it step into the lawn at the end of the street. From this point, you'll also get a fine view of North Beach far below.

Continue down the Vallejo St. steps to Taylor St., noting that photographer Dorothea Lange lived in an apartment at No. 1637 for several years during the late 1920s and early '30s. Cross Taylor and enter Ina Coolbrith Park, which like the steps you've just descended, stand in for

Diego Rivera's fresco

what would have been Vallejo St. if the hill hadn't been so steep. A plaque on a rock to the left of the park's entrance tells the story of Coolbrith, a poet who was named California's first poet laureate but is largely forgotten by today's literati. She is better remembered in Oakland, where she served as the city's first librarian. Meander down the steps, admiring the varying view as you lose altitude. At the bottom, you'll find yourself just a couple of blocks from the heart of North Beach—and at the end of this tour.

POINTS OF INTEREST

San Francisco Art Institute 800 Chestnut St., 415-771-7020

Bimbo's 365 Club 1025 Columbus Ave., 415-474-0365

route summary

1. Begin at the corner of Hyde and Lombard streets, and head down the curvy street.
2. Turn left on Leavenworth St.
3. Turn right on Chestnut St.
4. Turn right on Broadway for a look at Bimbo's, then turn around.
5. Turn right on Taylor St.
6. After crossing Union St., head up steps to Macondray Lane.
7. Turn left on Leavenworth St.
9. Turn left on Green St.
10. Turn right on Jones St.
11. Turn left on Vallejo St.
12. Follow steps down to Taylor St., cross Taylor, and continue down through Ina Coolbrith Park.

Bay windows and view of Alcatraz

Eddy St

Turk St

Turk St

Golden Gate Ave

Elm St

Polk St

Van Ness Ave

Larkin St

Hyde St

Leavenworth St

7th St

Redwood St

McAllister St

United Nations Plaza

City Hall

Civic Center Plaza

Fulton St

start

CIVIC CENTER

War Memorial Opera House

Grove St

finish

Grove St

Lech Walesa St

Polk St

Larkin St

Market St

8th St

Symphony Hall

Hayes St

Hayes St

Fox Plaza

9th St

Mission St

Van Ness Ave

Franklin St

Fell St

10th St

| 0 | 100 | 200 | 300 yards |
| 0 | 100 | 200 | 300 meters |

12 CIVIC Center: Beaux Arts Beauties and Cathedrals of Culture

BOUNDARIES: **Market St., Leavenworth St., McAllister St., Van Ness Ave.**
DISTANCE: **1 mile**
DIFFICULTY: **Easy**
PARKING: **There is an underground parking lot beneath Civic Center Plaza.**
PUBLIC TRANSIT: **Civic Center BART station; F streetcars; 5, 6, 9, 21, 31, and 71 Muni buses**

San Francisco's Civic Center is one of the most elegant and cohesively planned complexes in the U.S. Huge monumental Beaux Arts structures went up after the 1906 quake, making the area impressive but cold on the surface. Some of the buildings house offices of government, while others are pillars of high culture and contribute much-needed warmth to the neighborhood. The opera, the symphony, the Main Library, and the Asian Art Museum are all clustered around City Hall, which itself is one of the country's finest capitol buildings. The area is always busy, especially on weekdays when local, state, and federal government workers file in and out of the buildings along with museum goers and grade-school students bused in for field trips. On Wednesday and Sunday the farmers' market, going strong since 1981, adds even more life and diversity to the area, making these days ideal for a trek through the neighborhood.

● **Start at United Nations Plaza, at the corner of Market and Leavenworth. Named in commemoration of the 1945 signing of the United Nations Charter near here (see Herbst Theater, below), the plaza is a somewhat awkward open space that on most days merely serves as a shortcut from Market St. to the library and City Hall. The Heart of the City Farmers' Market changes that on Wednesday and Sunday, when vendors from Northern California farms set up stalls overflowing with produce, nuts, seafood, baked goods, and flowers. It's a lively and upbeat market that contrasts greatly with the usual down-and-outers who congregate around the plaza's fountain. From anywhere in the plaza, you can turn around and see Rigo's *Truth* mural emblazoned on the top floors of a Market St. building. Rigo painted the mural in 2002. U.N. Plaza was designed by Lawrence Halprin in the mid-1970s. An upcoming $100 million restoration of the landmark building at 50 U.N. Plaza will no doubt spark a resurgence of this vital walkway.**

● Pass through the plaza and cross Hyde St. Head west, up Fulton St., which separates the Main Library (to the left) and the Asian Art Museum (to the right). In the middle of the street stands the intriguing Pioneer Monument, commissioned by millionaire James Lick, who made his fortune by playing the real estate game in the Gold Rush city. Lick hired sculptor Frank Happersberger to create a tribute to the argonauts of that era. Thus, we have this large monument with bronze miners panning for gold beneath the bronze figure of the Roman goddess Minerva, standing on what appears to be a huge granite fire plug.

● The Asian Art Museum occupies the former main library, a beaux arts structure originally built in 1917. When the library moved into its current home across the street the old library building was remodeled—saving some of its luxuriant landmark features such as its lobby and stairway—to accommodate the immense holdings of the Asian Art Museum, which had outgrown its space in Golden Gate Park. The core of the collection was donated to the museum by Avery Brundage, the Chicago developer who also served as president of the International Olympic Committee for two decades. Brundage's huge bequest was the impetus for the founding of the museum and still comprises half the collection. Religious, military, and artistic objects span the entire region, from the Philippines to Iran, and some date back as far as 6,000 years. You can peek in at the lobby or have lunch in its cafe without paying the $12 general admission price.

● Retrace your steps and cross Fulton St. to the Main Library, which opened in 1995 to mostly positive reviews. Enter the building on the Larkin St. side and take an elevator to the fifth floor. From here, you can look down the building's central atrium, or climb to the top floor via Alice Aycock's spiral staircase, which ascends toward a fetching geometric glass ceiling. The library has many reading and research rooms that are worth perusing, including special collections with materials relating to the varied ethnic and cultural groups of San Francisco. The top floor is occupied by the excellent San Francisco History Center, which always has an informative exhibit of photos, newspaper clippings, and other items from its collection. Other thoughtful and interesting exhibits, some culled from the History Center collection, are in the Jewett Gallery, on the basement level of the library.

● Cross Larkin and walk through Civic Center Plaza toward the back of City Hall. The plaza is remarkable for its plainness and is often populated by homeless sunbathers. Sometimes you'll catch a large group of office workers participating in an organized tai chi exercise routine.

● On the Polk St. side of City Hall a statue of Abraham Lincoln appears ready to hold a discourse with anyone walking by. Head up the steps and enter City Hall, which is open to anyone not brandishing a firearm. San Francisco's City Hall has had a tumultuous past. Its predecessor, which stood where the Asian Art Museum is now, took two decades to build, and soon after its completion it crumbled to the ground in the initial temblor of 1906. It seems shady construction had resulted in a flimsy structure. All that remains is the head of the Goddess of Progress statue that stood atop the old city hall's dome (you'll see her in the South Wing exhibit). The current Beaux Arts City Hall was completed in 1915, and there is much to admire about it. The firm of Bakewell and Brown designed it. The dome, lovingly restored during Mayor Willie Brown's tenure, is taller than the Capitol dome in Washington, D.C. Wander the main floor to gaze up at the magnificent rotunda and at the staircase spilling down like the train of a bridal gown.

Tragedy came to City Hall in 1978, when Mayor George Moscone and Harvey Milk, the city's first gay supervisor, were shot and killed in their offices by former supervisor Dan White. White's lawyers convinced the jury that he was mentally instable, and on the night he was convicted of manslaughter rather than murder, outraged gays rioted in front of City Hall. The night is remembered as "White Night." On a lighter note, Marilyn Monroe and Joe DiMaggio were married in a civil ceremony in City Hall in 1954. So were some 4,000 same-sex couples in a startling display of civil disobedience in February 2004. Newly elected Mayor Gavin Newsom defied state law by permitting the weddings, and he even presided over some of the ceremonies. Gay brides and grooms lined out the doors of City Hall for weeks with an armada of media trucks clogging up traffic, creating a street-party atmosphere. Newsom was soon stopped, and the state revoked the unions, only to reverse its stance a few years later.

● After looking around City Hall, exit on the Van Ness side. Two nearly identical landmark buildings share the block across the street from City Hall. On the right (north side) is the War Memorial Veterans Building, which was designed by Bakewell and Brown and completed in 1932. Inside, the Herbst Theater is an intimate performance hall that gained renown in June 1945 when the United Nations Charter was signed in a ceremony on its stage. Off the front lobby, the San Francisco Arts Commission Gallery is a never-dull exhibition space for contemporary artists. Admission is free so take a look.

- From Veterans Hall mosey on over to the War Memorial Opera House. The two buildings, which commemorate the soldiers who fought in World War I, were built at the same time, and Arthur Brown Jr. (of Bakewell and Brown) designed the Opera House. G. Albert Lansburgh designed the Opera House's elegant interior. The San Francisco Opera was founded in 1923, and the opening night of each opera season is a big event among opera aficionados and socialites.

- At Grove St., Louise M. Davies Symphony Hall is a modern structure that looks its best on performance nights, when the curved glass facade is ablaze with warm light. The hall was built in 1980 and has housed the city's lauded symphony ever since. If you're a mite peckish or parched, Absinthe Brasserie and Bar is just around the corner, at Hayes and Franklin. It's a stylish recreation of a belle époque brasserie where you can slurp raw oysters or eat traditional French fare.

- Cross Van Ness and walk two blocks east on Grove. The Bill Graham Civic Auditorium faces Civic Center Plaza. Named for the legendary rock and roll impresario, Bill Graham, who based his operations in San Francisco, the auditorium is frequently the sight of performances by major rock artists. On the sidewalk in front of the building you'll stroll over a "Walk of Fame," embedded with plaques honoring local music figures.

POINTS OF INTEREST

Asian Art Museum 200 Larkin St., 415-581-3500

Main Library 100 Larkin St., 415-557-4400

San Francisco Arts Commission Gallery 401 Van Ness Ave., 415-554-6080

Absinthe Brasserie and Bar 398 Hayes St., 415-551-1590

ROUTE SUMMARY

1. Start at United Nations Plaza, at the corner of Market and Leavenworth streets.
2. Walk through U.N. Plaza toward Hyde St.
3. Cross Hyde St. and head up Fulton St.
4. Turn right at Larkin St., to the Asian Art Museum.
5. Retrace your steps and cross Fulton St. to visit the Main Library.
6. Cross Larkin St. and walk through Civic Center Plaza.
7. Cross Polk St. at Grove St. and enter City Hall through the building's east entrance.
8. Walk through City Hall and exit on the Van Ness side.
9. Turn right and cross Van Ness Ave. at McAllister St.
10. Turn left (on opposite side of Van Ness Ave.).
11. At Grove turn left.

San Francisco City Hall

Fern St

Hemlock St

Cedar St

Myrtle St

Olive St

Willow St

Sutter St

Leavenworth St

Hyde St

Post St

Post St

Cosmo Pl

Post St

finish

Geary St

Larkin St

Polk St

Geary St

O'Farrell St

Ellis St

Taylor St

Mason St

Hyde St

Ellis St

Leavenworth St

Jones St

Taylor St

Eddy St

Eddy St

Turk St

Van Ness Ave

Polk St

Turk St

Golden Gate Ave

Elm St

Golden Gate Ave

Redwood St

McAllister St

Larkin St

McAllister St

Market St

Stevenson St

6th St

Jessie St

United
Nations
Plaza

start

7th St

7th St

Mission St

Minna St

City Hall

Civic
Center
Plaza

Fulton St

CIVIC CENTER

0   100   200   300 yards

0   100   200   300 meters

13 TENDERLOIN: EARNING A FINER CUT

BOUNDARIES: **Market St, Taylor St, Post St, Polk St**
DISTANCE: **Approx. 1 mile**
DIFFICULTY: **Easy**
PARKING: **Street parking is metered, and not necessarily safe. There's a lot next to Original Joe's (corner of Taylor and Turk) and another at 550 O'Farrell St.**
PUBLIC TRANSIT: **Civic Center BART station; all Market St. buses and streetcars**

The Tenderloin, squeezed between Union Square and Civic Center, has long been the part of town where most of the city's lowlife ends up. It is block after block of Skid Rows lined mostly with residential hotels, rescue missions, and dive bars. Day and night, the sidewalks are crowded with the homeless and mentally ill, as well as a retinue of hustlers and drug dealers. It's all an unpleasant reminder that the American Dream doesn't quite pan out for everybody. That said, the Tenderloin is an incredibly interesting part of town that has intriguing history, good Vietnamese restaurants, inviting drinking establishments, and buildings that intimate compelling stories—stories perhaps in the Dashiell Hammett vein, for it was here the great crime writer penned his best works. The gay community has had a presence here for decades. Immigrants from Southeast Asia and the Middle East also live and do business in the T.L. Add to the mix a growing number of post-dot-com hipsters who favor the neighborhood's urban grit and the sophisticated nightclubs along Geary Ave. and Polk St.

● We'll start from U.N. Plaza on Market St. and head up Leavenworth into the 'Loin. On Golden Gate Ave., turn right and you'll spot St. Boniface Roman Catholic Church, built in 1906. Its German Romanesque style is a reflection of the immigrant parishioners of that time. Today St. Boniface, while still quite beautiful, is known more as a daytime refuge for the homeless, dozens of whom snooze in the pews from 6:30 a.m. to 2 p.m. Daily mass, funerals, and even weddings take place in the church to the accompaniment of a quiet chorus of snores. Church staff and the homeless of the T.L. call a nap here "sacred sleep." Sunday mass always livens the place up, and when the weather's nice parishioners sell homemade tamales in the church courtyard.

Past St. Boniface still heading east on Golden Gate Ave., ropes along the sidewalk lead around the corner to St. Anthony's Dining Room, where hot meals have been ladled out to the needy since 1950. The St. Anthony Foundation also provides clothing, housing, and medical care in a determined effort to "put ourselves out of business," as foundation literature puts it. SAF is over 100 years old now.

On the corner of Jones, a freshly painted mural honors the neighborhood and its history, depicting these streets from above with buildings demolished long ago drifting into the sky like ghostly balloons.

● Turn left at Taylor St., around the front of the Golden Gate Theatre. Across the street you'll see the back of the Warfield Theatre, where more murals pay homage to past performances and historic street scenes.

Taylor, you'll soon notice, has its share of seedy bars with colorful old signs (65 CLUB, 21 CLUB) suggesting these places may have come down a step or two in recent decades. The faded old logos would have looked snappy on cocktail napkins or matchbooks once upon a time. You'll encounter dozens of people sitting on the sidewalk and milling about, often speaking familiarly amongst each other, occasionally turning to a stranger for spare change or a dollar.

For a long time, the sole beacon on Taylor St. was Original Joe's. The friendly chef on Joe's neon sign still smiles down at passersby, but the sign itself is starting to fall apart. The restaurant has been shuttered since October 2007, when a fire gutted its plush dining room. The owners, the Duggan family, hope to reopen the restaurant, though they're looking at new locations in the city. Joe's, which had been around since 1937 and retained much of its traditional urban appeal up to the end, is sorely missed here. It was the last good place to go for an honest steak or a 3/4-pound charbroiled burger served on fresh sourdough bread. Joe's was a proud link to the district's workaday past. The Tenderloin supposedly derived its name, indirectly, from increased wages paid to local cops for walking a tough beat. Or perhaps cops here enjoyed opportunities for illicit income on the side. In any case, as the story goes, their wallets were somewhat fattened and they could afford better cuts of meat—the tender loins. Joe's was just the sort of place a flush cop might have dined. (Of course, this popular explanation pointedly fails to acknowledge the loins of the multitudes of high-skirted women who have walked these streets over the years, and who may also explain the district's name.)

● Double back to Turk St. and turn right. We'll pass Aunt Charlie's Lounge, at 133 Turk. It's the district's oldest gay bar and the entertainment here is of the "gender illusionist" and lip-syncing variety. The headliner is Gina La Divina, who cheerfully bills herself as the $65,000 Silicon Wonder. She has been performing in Frisco since the 1970s but doesn't look a day over 40, give or take a decade or two.

● Along the next couple of uneventful blocks of Turk you'll pass a huge Salvation Army headquarters, a senior center or two, and a little junk shop called Krim Kram's Bargain Mart. The Turk-Hyde Mini-Park, a rare public space in the Tenderloin, fills a lot where an apartment building once stood. Also on the Turk-Hyde corner, a vacant parking lot is a poor substitute for the legendary Blackhawk nightclub, which once occupied the site. On this spot, in April 1961, Miles Davis' quintet recorded the celebrated live album *Friday and Saturday Night Miles Davis in Person at the Blackhawk, San Francisco.* (It's still available in a four-disc box set.)

● Turn right and continue on Hyde St. for a block. You'll pass the dowdy looking Lafayette Coffee Shop, with signs promising PRIME RIB (in neon) and FINE FOOD (in stenciled paint), but the place looks like it has been festering in its own grease for decades. Next door the Cadillac Market, selling package liquors and processed foods, seems to suggest at least one Detroit icon still has a little cache somewhere. The Brown Jug, on the opposite corner, is a dive that has found new life serving a younger, hipper crowd.

● Hang a Louie at Eddy St., endure an uninteresting block, and you'll soon spot the Phoenix Hotel, on the corner of Larkin. It's a classic mid-20th-century motel, with parking, two levels of rooms, and a kidney-shaped pool—but over the past two decades it's become much more than that. When in San Francisco, rock stars and younger movie stars tend to sleep here. Nirvana, Keanu Reeves, Norah Jones, David Bowie, and countless others have parted the sheets here. Those who sleep at the Phoenix may be tempted to gravitate to the attached Bambuddha Lounge, a glamour-puss magnate that seems to have a knack for making ordinary patrons feel unwelcome.

Directly across the street from the Bambuddha, the somewhat drab apartment building at 620 Eddy was the home of author Dashiell Hammett, who lived here with his wife and two daughters from mid-1921 until mid-1926. Hammett was not well known at the time, but he published many of his Continental Op stories, about an unnamed gumshoe, while living here. (We'll see Hammett's next home in just a few blocks.)

● Rather than heading any farther up Eddy, turn right on Larkin St. and pass through the portals to Little Saigon, a two-block concentration of Southeast Asian restaurants and shops. Mangosteen and Vietnam II are highly regarded, and there are a number of other intriguing holes-in-the-walls for inexpensive noodles and sandwiches. For many, Little Saigon is the Tenderloin's only allure.

● Turn left on Ellis St. and right on Polk St. Here we enter Polk Gulch, world renowned for the gay scene that formed here during the 1970s. (Polk St. was the decidedly less refined flip side of the Castro.) At Olive Alley a huge whale mural comes into view. It tattoos the backside of the Mitchell Brothers O'Farrell Theater, a true landmark in the neighborhood. Along the Polk St. side of the building, an even more eye-catching jungle mural extends the entire block with leopards, tigers, and gorillas lurking in the shadows. Very likely, the mural is meant to suggest the wild sexuality going on within the theater, which can be accessed at 895 O'Farrell St. The theater opened in 1969 and is where Artie and Jim Mitchell screened the low-budget pornographic films they made. The duo gained notoriety with such porn classics as *Behind the Green Door*, starring Marilyn Chambers. The Mitchell Brothers' empire grew to include 11 theaters throughout California. In 1991 Jim shot and killed Artie, copped a manslaughter conviction, and served six years in jail. Nevertheless, the theater, long ago converted into a live strip club, is considered one of the city's classiest venues for exotic dancing. A couple of doors down, the Great American Music Hall is a former bordello that's surprisingly posh inside. It's an excellent live-music venue that books quality touring acts several nights a week.

● Continue on Polk and turn right at Geary St. You might be tempted to stop for a pint of Fullers or a dram of Laphroig at Edinburgh Castle, but let's hold that thought for future reference. The huge old pub is worth noting for its cultural contribution to the neighborhood and the city at large. Manager Alan Black, a man with an admirable fondness for working-class literature, has turned the pub's upstairs room into a theater where plays, live music, and readings are performed. Black and his partners also run a publishing house. Irvine Welsh, author of *Trainspotting,* has made several appearances at the pub, where he has read from his work and witnessed a dramatic adaptation of *Trainspotting*. Welsh took a liking to San Francisco and moved to the city in 2003.

● Continue on Geary, noting some of the historic old dives, such as the Ha Ra, which opened way back in 1947. The Gangway, a few doors up Larkin St., is an old gay bar with an obvious sailor theme—the rickety bow of the *Titanic* juts out from the façade. The next couple of blocks of Geary are transitional. The street is graced by some elegant early-20th-century apartment buildings, such as the Castle Apartments, along with a Hispanic bodega burgeoning with fresh fruit carts out on the sidewalk, and, across the street, the trendy Cairo Nights hookah lounge.

● At Hyde St, turn left, then pause at the corner of Post. The very smart-looking apartment building at 891 Post was home to Hammett at least from late 1927 through the end of 1928. He may have lived here even longer, as a plaque on the side of the building suggests. It is very likely that Hammett wrote *Red Harvest* and *Dain Curse* while living here, and he probably drafted *The Maltese Falcon* in the apartment as well. Literary sleuths like Don Herron, reading *Falcon* very closely, have deduced that Sam Spade's apartment must have been in this building.

　　At the other end of this block, Kayo Books sells old paperback mysteries and sleazy fiction from the '50s and '60s—it's a fun little shop and a true homage to the neighborhood's history and culture.

● Make a right at Leavenworth St., then turn left on Geary for a look at the fantastic Alcazar Theater. Built for the Shriners in 1917, and designed by T. Patterson Ross (himself a Shriner), the theater is meant to evoke Byzantine grandeur with intricate archways clad in ornate tiles. You'll notice some familiar motifs—above a second story window on the far right look for a Shriner fez.

● From here, head on down Geary to Union Square, or go around the block for a fine vegetarian Vietnamese meal at Golden Era Vegetarian Restaurant, on O'Farrell St. The food and atmosphere are top-notch.

POINTS OF INTEREST

Aunt Charlie's Lounge 133 Turk St., 415-441-2922

Phoenix Hotel 601 Eddy St., 415-776-1380

Bambuddha Lounge 601 Eddy St., 415-885-5088

Mangosteen 601 Larkin St., 415-776-3999

Vietnam II 701 Larkin St., 415-885-1274

Mitchell Bros. O'Farrell Theater 895 O'Farrell St., 415-776-6686

Great American Music Hall 859 O'Farrell St., 415-885-0750

Edinburgh Castle 950 Geary St., 415-885-4074

Ha Ra 875 Geary St., 415-673-3148

Gangway 841 Larkin St., 415-776-6828

Kayo Books 814 Post St., 415-749-0554

Golden Era Vegetarian Restaurant 572 O'Farrell St., 415-673-3136

ROUTE SUMMARY

1. Begin at the corner of Market and Leavenworth streets and head north to Golden Gate Ave. and turn right.
2. Turn left on Taylor St.
3. Turn left on Turk St.
4. Turn right on Hyde St.
5. Turn left on Eddy St.
6. Turn right on Larkin St.
7. Turn left on Ellis St.
8. Turn right on Polk St.
9. Turn right on Geary St.
10. Turn left on Hyde St.
11. Turn right on Leavenworth St.
12. Turn left on Geary St.

O'Farrell Theater marquee

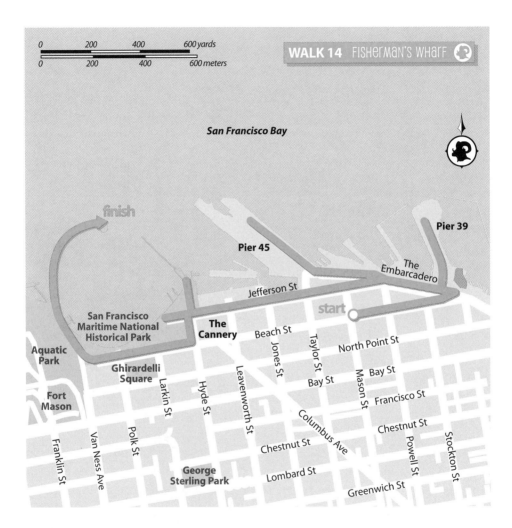

0   200   400   600 yards
0   200   400   600 meters

San Francisco Bay

finish

Pier 39

Pier 45

The Embarcadero

Jefferson St

start

San Francisco Maritime National Historical Park

The Cannery

Beach St

North Point St

Aquatic Park

Ghirardelli Square

Larkin St

Hyde St

Leavenworth St

Jones St

Taylor St

Bay St

Mason St

Bay St

Francisco St

Fort Mason

Franklin St

Van Ness Ave

Polk St

Columbus Ave

Chestnut St

Chestnut St

Powell St

Stockton St

George Sterling Park

Lombard St

Greenwich St

14 FISHERMAN'S WHARF: WHEN IN ROME, DO AS THE TOURISTS FROM YPSILANTI, MICHIGAN, DO

BOUNDARIES: **Beach St., Jefferson St., Grant Ave., Aquatic Park**
DISTANCE: **2½ miles**
DIFFICULTY: **Easy**
PARKING: **Off-street parking is available at Anchorage Square, corner of Leavenworth and Beach streets. Most street parking is metered seven days a week. On side streets south of Bay St. you might find unmetered street parking, limited to two hours for non-residents (on Sunday you can park for an unlimited time in these zones).**
PUBLIC TRANSIT: **Powell-Mason cable car; F streetcar; 47 Muni bus**

Nothing against tourists from Ypsilanti, mind you. But Fisherman's Wharf is the prototypical tourist trap, and for that reason most San Franciscans regard the neighborhood as a party that they haven't been invited to, and that they wouldn't want to attend anyway. But to go on deliberately avoiding this cash cow of a neighborhood is to lack curiosity.

For the most part the attractions here fail to reward an ironic approach, although, for some, it helps to be cloaked in such armor. A genuine appreciation for the city's maritime history will go much further. Here and there you'll also encounter aged remnants of Fisherman's Wharf's origins as a tourist trap—old boats, seafood stalls, and family-owned restaurants that opened way back in the 1930s. None of this is to suggest that after taking this tour you're likely to make a habit of spending time down here. But after separating wheat from chaff, you're sure to agree the neighborhood yields a surprising bounty.

● **Start at the Longshoremen's Hall, a homely but historic structure at the corner of Mason and Beach streets. It houses the headquarters of the International Longshoremen's and Warehousemen's Union. Bodies outlined on the sidewalk suggest this corner was a crime scene, but these figures are tributes to the striking longshoremen who were shot by police in the general strike of 1934. The riot and shootings took place not here, but on the corner of Mission and Steuart streets, where the Coast Seamen's Union kept its offices. A significant historic event did take place in this building in January 1966, when the Trips Festival was held here.**

The three-day event, organized by Ken Kesey (who penned *One Flew Over the Cuckoo's Nest*), rock promoter Bill Graham, and others, ushered in the hippie era. Entertainment was provided by the Grateful Dead, Big Brother and the Holding Company, light shows, and a "stroboscopic trampolinist" who hopped up and down while a strobe light flickered on him. The real point of the festival was to drop acid, and some 6,000 people showed up to do just that. Take a look through the plate-glass windows and imagine the place full of wigged-out hippies.

● Turn right onto Beach St., which hits Jefferson St. Cross Jefferson to enter Pier 39. This open-air shopping center is about as touristy as it gets, with businesses obviously preying upon impulsive shoppers. Head straight to the San Francisco Carousel, a handcrafted classic, made in Italy. Horses and chariots rotate around a mechanical organ in the center. Rides cost $3. Also pay a visit to K Dock, at the pier's western side, where a small colony of California sea lions overtook a row of boat docks in 1990. The colony quickly grew, and now as many as 900 barking sea lions compete for space on the docks on a winter's day. In summer, most of them migrate to warmer waters to breed, but a few usually haul out here year-round. They're rightly the biggest attraction on Pier 39.

● Exiting the pier, turn right onto Jefferson St. and walk two blocks until you see and smell the Boudin Bakery. The modern building is nothing much to look at, but the company has been providing the city with sourdough bread since 1849, and some of its "mother dough" is said to have been carried over from the first batch. No need to stop, unless you want a snack.

● Veer right, onto Pier 45. The sight of a submarine and a liberty ship from World War II will tell you you're on the right track. The submarine is USS *Pampanito,* which patrolled the Pacific during the latter half of the war. You can board the sub to see how uncomfortable life beneath the waves must have been, and to puzzle over the state-of-the art technology of a bygone era. The liberty ship is SS *Jeremiah O'Brien,* a cargo-carrying vessel that delivered supplies to Normandy on D-Day. It's fully outfitted and in working order. Board and head straight for the engine room for an astonishing view of the ship's awesome 2,700-horsepower, triple-expansion steam engine. *Steamboy* fans will be in heaven.

Also on Pier 45, the Musée Mécanique is the hidden gem of Fisherman's Wharf. For some, it's the only excuse to venture into this part of town. It's the private collection of Edward Galland Zelinsky, consisting of mechanical amusements and games, mostly from the early 20th century. Risqué mutoscope moving pictures (mostly of women showing their ankles), player pianos, and old-fashioned black-and-white photo booths will easily suck the quarters out of your pockets. Save a few coins for the real showstoppers—"automata" displays of carnivals and circuses, toothpick Ferris wheels, and even a Chinese opium den with a dragon that peeps out from behind a curtain. Be sure to pump some quarters into Laffin' Sal to keep her howling. Her belly laughs are infectious. Some of the one-of-a-kind machines here are fine works of folk art.

About an hour later, as you reemerge into the real world, head directly back toward Jefferson St. On the way you'll pass the oldest seafood restaurants in the district. Fishermen's Grotto No. 9 was the postcard establishment of the local tourism industry about half a century ago. It opened in 1935 and is still owned by the Geraldi family. Inside you'll find a swanky mid-century bar that's not always open. There's also a gift shop that includes some dusty old relics that have probably sat on the shelves for several decades. Most of the seafood restaurants on the wharf are named for Italian families, reflecting the traditional preeminence of Italian fishermen in the local seafood industry. The families of fishermen often ran little seafood stalls to augment their income, and these eventually became restaurants. Most of the restaurants still operate sidewalk stalls selling boiled crab and clam chowder served up in hollowed out loaves of sourdough bread. These are your best bet if you're hungry.

An iconic Fisherman's Wharf restaurant

● Turn right at Jefferson St. Behind Fishermen's Grotto some very charming and collectible leisure craft—wooden two-seaters mostly—are moored. A block down at Jefferson and Leavenworth, is the Cannery, an old Del Monte plant that was converted into a shopping center in 1968. The old brick plant was built in 1907 for the Fruit Packers Association, which packed fruit and produce grown in the Central Valley. A courtyard that separates the Cannery from the brick Haslett Warehouse is a nice space where a few restaurants and a bar have tables on the patio and musicians perform around lunchtime. Jack's Cannery serves decent pub grub here.

In the Haslett Warehouse, on the corner of Jefferson and Hyde streets, the Maritime Visitor Center is a gateway to the shipping history that more or less takes over this tour. There's a beautiful antique lighthouse glass set up in front, affording a rare up-close look. The bulk of the space here is dedicated to generally excellent exhibits of art and archival material that tell the story of the seafarers and explorers who passed through the Golden Gate. Entry is free. Upstairs, the Haslett Warehouse has been converted into the boutique Argonaut Hotel.

● Across Jefferson, the entry to Hyde St. Pier is obvious, thanks to a large sign spanning the pier. You'll also quickly spot the fleet of 19th-century ships tied up here. These include *Balclutha,* a square-rigger that regularly traveled the route around Cape Horn from San Francisco to Europe; *Alma,* a graceful flat-bottomed scow that transported grain to communities around San Francisco Bay; and *C.A. Thayer,* a three-masted schooner that carried lumber up and down the Pacific Coast. There are many more vessels and items of interest here, and visitors are free to casually explore them. The pier itself was a ferry launch for Route 101 automobile traffic until the Golden Gate Bridge was completed in 1937. Admission is $5.

● Hyde St. Pier flanks one side of Aquatic Park, which slopes down to a narrow crescent of sand. A sidewalk leads from the pier round the beach, where you'll spot hearty swimmers braving the icy cold waters of the bay.

● Rather than round the beach, though, cut straight out on Hyde St. (We'll make our way back to the water in a few minutes.) The Buena Vista Cafe, at the corner of Hyde and Beach, overlooks the park. It's one of San Francisco's classic saloons, having opened in 1916 in an old boarding house. The place stakes its reputation on having introduced Irish coffee to the U.S. in 1952, and there's usually a row of glasses lined up on the bar awaiting hot coffee, a jigger of Irish whiskey, and a dollop of whipped cream. On a clammy San Francisco day, it's what the doctor ordered.

● Turn right on Beach St. and you'll soon reach Ghirardelli Square, where the Ghirardelli Chocolate Co. moved to from its former location in Jackson Square (see the Barbary Coast walk). The red-brick Chocolate Building was completed in 1899, and as the company grew, founder Domingo Ghirardelli's sons added the Cocoa Building (1900), the Clock Tower (1911), and the Power House (1915). The huge sign atop the complex is one of San Francisco's most recognizable landmarks. The company moved its operations to the East Bay in the early 1960s, and the complex reopened as a shopping center in 1964.

● At the corner of Beach and Polk streets, overlooking Aquatic Park, is the San Francisco National Maritime Museum. It is appropriately housed in the Art Deco Sala Burton Building shaped like a steamship, replete with port holes. It was a public bath house and a casino before being repurposed for the Maritime Museum. The museum is currently undergoing restoration—"in drydock" as the old salts who run it like to say—though it is possible to enter the lobby to see Hilaire Hiler's whimsical floor-to-ceiling mural depicting a trippy underwater scene. There are some interesting sculptures by Beniamino Bufano and an abstract mosaic work by Sargent Johnson on the veranda. If the museum is closed, you can still admire Johnson's green slate carvings around the front entrance.

● From the Maritime Museum, make your way back toward the beach and turn left onto the walkway, which will lead to the eyelash-shaped Municipal Pier, which gets you out into the bay without a boat.

POINTS OF INTEREST

Boudin Bakery **160 Jefferson St., 415-928-1849**

USS *Pampanito* **Pier 45, 415-561-7006**

SS *Jeremiah O'Brien* **Pier 45, 415-544-0100**

Musée Mécanique **Pier 45 Shed A, 415-346-2000**

Fisherman's Grotto No 9 **9 Fisherman's Wharf, 415-673-7025**

Maritime Visitor Center **Hyde and Jefferson Sts., 415-447-5000**

Argonaut Hotel **495 Jefferson St., 415-563-0800**

Hyde St. Pier **415-447-5000**

Buena Vista Cafe **2765 Hyde St., 415-474-5044**

San Francisco National Maritime Museum **900 Beach St., 415-561-7100**

ROUTE SUMMARY

1. Start at the corner of Mason and Beach streets.
2. Head three blocks east (right) on Beach St. and turn left onto Jefferson St.
3. Cross Jefferson St. and enter Pier 39.
4. Go to the San Francisco Carousel, and then to K Dock to see the sea lions before exiting back onto Jefferson St.
5. Follow Jefferson St. 2.5 blocks and turn right onto Pier 45.
6. Exit Pier 45 and walk past the Fisherman's Grotto No. 9 back to Jefferson St.
7. Turn right and follow Jefferson St. two blocks to the Cannery.
8. Cross Jefferson St to enter Hyde St. Pier.
9. Exit Hyde St. Pier and cut over to the corner of Hyde and Beach streets and turn right on Beach St.
10. Past the Maritime Museum, at Polk St., turn right to sidewalk that follows the curve of the beach.
11. Follow the curve onto the Municipal Pier and walk all the way to the pier's end.

The Balclutha

0   200   400   600 yards
0   200   400   600 meters

San Francisco Bay

start

Marina Green

Marina Blvd

Jefferson St

Beach St   Beach St

Fillmore St

Webster St

Buchanan St

Laguna St

Fort Mason

Bay St

Francisco St

Van Ness Ave

Palace of Fine Arts

Broderick St

Baker St

Bay St

Scott St

Avila St

Pierce St

Octavia St

Chestnut St

Lombard St

Greenwich St

Franklin St

101

Chestnut St

Webster St

Buchanan St

Filbert St

Union St

finish

Gough St

Lombard St

Greenwich St

The Presidio

Lyon St

Baker St

Broderick St

Divisadero St

Filbert St

Union St

Green St

Pierce St

Steiner St

Fillmore St

Green St

Vallejo St

Broadway

Laguna St

Octavia St

15 MARINA AND COW HOLLOW: SWINGIN' IN THE URBAN JUNGLE GYM WITH WELL-TO-DO YOUNGSTERS

BOUNDARIES: **Van Ness Ave., Baker St., Green St., and San Francisco Bay**
DISTANCE: **3½ miles**
DIFFICULTY: **Easy**
PARKING: **Off-street parking in Fisherman's Wharf is your best bet.**
PUBLIC TRANSIT: **Powell-Hyde cable car; 30, 47 Muni buses**

The Marina might be summed up as the new-money counterpart to old-money Pacific Heights. Both are upper-class enclaves, but while Pacific Heights rises above the city with a Victorian regalness, the Marina thrusts its chest out into the bay with a 20th-century brashness. Cow Hollow, being neither up the hill nor along the bay, more or less slides into the Marina, and the two neighborhoods feel like two parts of a whole. Single professionals have been drawn to the area since the yuppies of the 1980s claimed the neighborhood. You'll encounter young urban professionals throughout the city, but those of the Marina and Cow Hollow still seem to be of their own special stripe. The districts are remarkably mainstream, at least by San Francisco standards. The city's countercultural leanings are little felt here. On this walk, we'll set out to appreciate the Marina's location with a brisk hike along the bayfront, then loop back down the commercial Main Streets of both neighborhoods.

●   Start at Aquatic Park, just beyond the end of Van Ness, where a paved footpath follows the curve of a rare bayside beachfront. Follow the path toward (but not onto) the eyelash-shaped pier, then go left on McDowell Rd. and follow the ramp up to Fort Mason. (The Fort Mason GGNRA sign will tell you you're on the right track.) At Bunker Rd., behind the youth hostel, double back up the two-track dirt road, which leads to the 1863 Battery. Perhaps you'll feel safe in this shady spot armed with a Civil War–era cannon. So far, the cannon has never been fired in hostility. Let's hope it stays that way. This promontory became a defensive battery way back in 1797, when the Spanish established the Battery San Jose here.

- Follow the trail past the cannon and some picnic tables, and then go up some concrete steps. At the top of the steps, a concrete path leads into the residential part of Fort Mason. The fine Victorians along the east side of Franklin St. were originally built for civilians. Although the land was always owned by the military, as the city grew quickly in the 1850s developers went ahead and built homes here, in what was then known as Black Point. It was a gamble worth taking, for the front row views of the bay from the bluffs here are spectacular. Eventually, these homes housed military officers. The last building on the left, at the corner of Pope St. and MacArthur Ave., is the Officers' Club.

- Nothing against officers, but head in the opposite direction. You'll soon reach the visitor center, where you can grab maps and literature for future visits to the Golden Gate National Recreation Area, of which Fort Mason is a part. Past it, look for the blacktop path that wends through the green of the Great Meadow. In one corner, before a grassy amphitheater, a statue of the late Congressman Phillip Burton appears to be orating. Burton chaired a subcommittee on national parks and increased the amount of protected parkland in the United States during the late 1970s.

- Follow the path through the Great Meadow until tile roofs to the northwest come into view. Head in that direction and you'll find a sign that says "piers," with an arrow pointing down. That's the idea. You'll see the steps, which lead to the lower half of Fort Mason. Three piers and five whitewashed wooden warehouses remain from what was the U.S.'s largest embarkation port on the Pacific from the Spanish-American War on through to World War II. These piers and sheds were built by 1915. During the 1960s, as the military began shutting the fort down, Congressman Burton set his sights on creating a national park, the GGNRA, to include these scenic bluffs and historic buildings. The sheds today house an assortment of cultural institutions, including the renowned Magic Theatre, which has premiered works by Sam Shepard and David Mamet, among others. Also here is Greens, one of the more famous vegetarian restaurants in the country. Affiliated with the Zen Center of San Francisco, Greens opened in 1979. If it's mealtime, you can grab a healthy sack lunch and find a spot on the piers for a picnic. Also while here, take a look inside SFMoMA's Artists' Gallery, where works by contemporary artists are exhibited and sold. Then duck into Book Bay Fort Mason, where the Friends of the San Francisco Public Library sell off the SFPL's cast-off and donated books and movies at bargain prices.

From Fort Mason, an asphalt path rounds a small yacht harbor before meeting the sidewalks of the Marina Green, a long, gusty lawn along the bayshore that's perfect for kite flying. As the flatness of the terrain here makes apparent, much of the Marina is landfill, created shortly before and directly after the 1906 quake. Some of the fill is said to be rubble from buildings toppled during the quake, which is ironic, considering buildings on landfill are particularly vulnerable during earthquakes. Liquefaction occurs as the earth beneath the streets is shaken, turning the ground beneath foundations into jelly. This was cruelly borne out during the 1989 Loma Prieta earthquake, which inflicted more damage on the Marina than on any other part of the city.

The Marina Green is a long, uneventful stretch, so just enjoy the view and the exercise. The sailing craft moored in the harbor here belong to members of the exclusive St. Francis Yacht Club, founded in 1927, and the Golden Gate Yacht Club, founded 12 years later. The landfill and the harbor here were completed in time for the 1915 Panama Pacific Exhibition, which ostensibly celebrated the opening of the Panama Canal. Of course, the fair also demonstrated the reemergence of San Francisco, just nine years after the city was laid to waste, and it promoted the new patch of real estate that would soon become the Marina District. Strange and exotic buildings covered much of the fairgrounds, only to be torn down immediately afterward. The Mediterranean-style housing you see here now mostly went up in the 1920s.

The Marina Green sidles along Marina Blvd. for several blocks. At Baker St. turn right and then right again onto Yacht Rd. Follow the road all the way to the end to reach the Wave Organ, an unusual example of environmental art. Built by Peter

Fort Mason housing

Richards and George Gonzales in 1986, the Wave Organ is constructed of PVC pipe and busted headstones salvaged from a dismantled graveyard. The idea is to appreciate the sounds created by the tides passing through the pipes. Press an ear against the listening tubes that poke up out of the cobblestones—each one sounds different. The rumbling tones have a profound hush, like an amplified seashell. There's even a stereo booth, with various sounds coming at you from several tubes. The Wave Organ sounds best during high tide, which sometimes occurs at an unaccommodating time of day. (Check the website www.saltwatertides.com to see a tidal timetable for the day of your walk.) At lower tides, the sound emanating from the tubes resembles the chugging and wheezing of an old toilet. Still, it's unusual enough to warrant an out-of-the-way sidetrip.

● Return to Marina Blvd. and turn left on Baker St. A block up, the stately pillars of Bernard Maybeck's Palace of Fine Arts reflect off a duck pond. The palace, designed to look like a gutted classical ruin, is the only architectural showpiece spared after the Panama Pacific Exhibition. The original, made of plaster and chicken wire, wasn't designed to last, but it was faithfully rebuilt of durable concrete in the 1960s. Behind it, a shed from the fair also survives and houses the Exploratorium, a fun science museum.

● Stay on Baker until you reach Chestnut St., where a left turn leads into a fashionable shopping strip. Here, it may suddenly dawn on you that the Marina is the Beverly Hills of San Francisco, where everyone looks like a celebrity and some actually are. Among the expensive clothiers and training centers are a handful of spots to grab a cup of coffee or a bite to eat. Bechelli's is a classic coffee shop with swivel stools around a horseshoe counter. It has that traditional Main Street feel and the basic menu you'd expect in such a place. A few blocks up, Lucca Delicatessen has all the hallmarks of a great Italian deli, with the aroma of salamis and cheeses luring you in. There's a park ahead, if you want to grab a sandwich to go.

● At Fillmore St. turn right. After crossing busy Lombard St. you enter Cow Hollow. A block down, the Balboa Cafe welcomes you to the neighborhood. It's a great old bar and grill, open since 1913, with an interior that would look right at home in an Edward Hopper painting. Over lunch, you can enjoy the place for its historic atmosphere, but at night the neighborhood's noisy singles scene engulfs it. It was on the yuppie socialite map during the 1980s and remains hot today. Before he was mayor, Gavin Newsom, himself more a young urban entrepreneur (a "yueie"?), once owned it.

- Turn left on Filbert. At the corner of Webster St. the Vedanta Temple is one of the most exotic-looking places of worship in San Francisco. The Victorian pile is a purple flight of fancy with Moorish arches and turrets. It was built in 1905 by the Swami Trigunatitananda, the Hindu monk who founded the Vedanta Society of Northern California. Every tower is different—notice the medieval battlement atop one. Turn the corner to admire it from all sides.

- A block down Webster make a left on Union St., the main drag. Union is, you might say, visually busier than Chestnut St., with tighter clothes, bigger hairstyles, and bars that attract singles. Perry's, at No. 1944, has the feel of an old New York tavern, and indeed the bar was moved to here from the Upper East Side in 1969. Most of the time it's a casual neighborhood joint where you can watch a few innings of baseball over a beer and a burger. Late at night, though, Perry's is the archetypical "breeder" bar. ("Breeder," in SF's gay-conscious way of looking at things, is a straight person, particularly one who is single and sexually active.)

- Turn right on Gough for a look at the Colonial Dames Octagon House, at No. 2645. It was built in 1861. See the Russian Hill tour for background on unusual eight-sided houses such as this one. Next to it is a wooded park surrounded by an unpainted picket fence—a good spot to get off your feet after a long walk. Van Ness Ave. is just two blocks away.

POINTS OF Interest

Greens **Fort Mason Center, Building A, 415-771-6222**

Book Bay Fort Mason **Fort Mason Center, Building C, 415-771-1076**

Exploratorium **3601 Lyon St., 415-563-7337**

Bechelli's **2346 Chestnut St., 415-346-1801**

Lucca Delicatessen **2120 Chestnut St., 415-921-7873**

Balboa Cafe **3199 Fillmore St., 415-921-3944**

Vedanta Temple **2963 Webster St.**

Perry's **1944 Union St., 415-922-9022**

Colonial Dames Octagon House **2645 Gough St., 415-441-7512**

route summary

1. Start at the northern end of Van Ness Ave. and follow the path in a northwesterly direction around Aquatic Park.

2. Before you reach the pier, turn left on McDowell Ave.

3. Follow the path up the hill into Fort Mason.

4. Behind the youth hostel, turn left onto the two-track dirt road.

5. Past the cannon and picnic tables, follow steps up. A path will lead from the top of the steps to Pope St. residences.

6. Turn right on MacArthur Ave.

7. At the Great Meadow, follow the curving path to the right.

8. At the northern side of the meadow, look for the sign that says PIERS, pointing down steps that lead to the piers and warehouses of Fort Mason Center.

9. Past Fort Mason Center, turn right onto an asphalt path that hems the boat harbor.

10. Follow the sidewalk west, through the Marina Green.

11. Turn right at Baker St.

12. Turn right at Yacht Rd. and follow it to the Wave Organ, at the end.

13. Return to Baker St. and head south.

14. Turn left on Chestnut St.

15. Turn right on Fillmore St.

16. Turn left on Filbert St.

17. Turn right on Webster St.

18. Turn left on Union St.

19. Turn right on Gough St.

Vedanta Temple

WALK 16 Presidio

Golden Gate Bridge

Fort Point

San Francisco Bay

Coastal Trail

Toll Plaza

101

Crissy Field

start

finish

Allen St

Doyle

Palace of Fine Arts

Mason St

Lincoln Blvd

Sheridan Ave

Anza St

Lincoln Ave

Gorgas Ave

Letterman Digital Arts Center

Fort Winfield Scott

San Francisco National Cemetery

Mesa St

Dewitt Rd

Arguello Blvd

Portola St

Clark St

Presidio Blvd

The Presidio

Park Blvd

Pacific Ave

0   300   600   900 yards
0   300   600   900 meters

16 Presidio: Baywatching and Invading Old Forts

BOUNDARIES: **Crissy Field, Golden Gate Bridge, Letterman Complex**
DISTANCE: **5½ miles**
DIFFICULTY: **Moderate (but long)**
PARKING: **Free parking is available in several lots along Crissy Field.**
PUBLIC TRANSIT: **The 30 Muni bus terminates on Broderick St., a block outside the park, near Crissy Field.**

The Presidio, along with Mission Dolores, was just about all there was to San Francisco during the city's Spanish period. It was the Spanish military outpost, linked to the mission via a trail that later became Divisadero St. Its location overlooking the Golden Gate was suitable for guarding the entrance to San Francisco Bay. The Presidio's 1,000 acres remained a military outpost under the Mexican government. Under U.S. rule, the Presidio was an Army base until 1994, when it was turned over to the National Park System. As a park, it has a lot to offer. Its historic buildings include one of the city's very oldest structures, as well as many buildings from the Civil War period. Some rows of military housing built in the Colonial Revival style resemble a Norman Rockwell vision of small town American life, with wide porches and plenty of red brick and white trim. San Francisco's most recognizable architectural feature, the Golden Gate Bridge, touches down on the park's northern tip.

Meanwhile, post-military tenants of the park include George Lucas, whose film production companies are based here, and numerous non-profit organizations. But its the land and the location that make the Presidio special, for during its two centuries as a military base the area was spared the rapid development that went on outside its walls. Thus, an extraordinary swath of nature has been preserved for the leisurely enjoyment of the modern civilian. It is a huge and varied parkland, with cliffside trails overlooking the Pacific Ocean and a long, low-lying bayshore that draws walkers and bikers in great numbers. This tour is lengthy (over 5 miles) but doesn't even cover half the park. Regard it as an introduction to the key sights, and come back to explore the park further on your own.

● Start at Crissy Field, where San Franciscans come to appreciate their bay, and walk in the direction of the Golden Gate Bridge. The level grassy strip to the left was an airfield, formed by the Army in 1919. These were fairly early days in the development of flight, and many landmark voyages took off or landed here, including test runs at transcontinental flights. (Then, it took three days to make it from here to New York, with numerous pit stops along the way—not unlike a cross-country trip by Greyhound bus today.) In 1924, the first round-the-world journey by air made a heroic stop at Crissy Field before concluding at its starting point in Seattle, Washington. Two of the four aircraft that began the journey made it to the finish. The other two crashed. It was a dangerous endeavor for the times. The runway is said to be intact, but only kites and Frisbees take off here these days.

● Along the cinder path you'll see marshlands that are being restored to their pre-Army state. The marshes are home to great blue herons, great egrets, and double-crested cormorants, and attract plenty of migrating surf scoters, Caspian terns, and western grebes. It's busier than an international airport.

● Just beyond Crissy Field is the Warming Hut, a welcoming gift shop and snack stand that serves up hot beverages and high-quality sandwiches made with local and organic ingredients.

● Continue along the bayfront to Fort Point, with the Golden Gate Bridge arching dramatically overhead. Along the way, take note of steps heading uphill to the left (we'll walk up there in a bit). Also check out the seawall, where Kim Novak took her dip into the bay in Hitchcock's *Vertigo*. (She was fully clothed, and James Stewart leapt in after her, took her to his apartment, and managed to get her into a bathrobe without violating the strict film code.) On some days you'll see surfers riding the waves just off the point. Fort Point itself, a huge brick and granite fortress, was built in 1853 to protect the entrance to the bay. Construction continued through the Civil War, when it was thought a Confederate attack might arrive by sea. Many other buildings rose in the Presidio during that time, as San Francisco's importance became clear to the vulnerable Union. From Fort Point the perspective of the Golden Gate Bridge—from underneath it—will knock your socks off. The graceful immensity of the bridge fully registers here.

- Backtrack toward the Warming Hut and follow those steps we passed earlier. Toward the top, bear right on the trail that leads to Battery East. Built in 1876, this armed lookout is one of many built in the latter half of the 19th century along the bluffs overlooking the Pacific. Continue on the trail, which passes beneath the bridge toll plaza and by a few more historic batteries before reaching a coastal overlook (just beyond Battery Godfrey). From the overlook, follow Langdon Ct., which loops to Lincoln Blvd., and cross over to Fort Winfield Scott. This complex, built in 1910, has many Mission Revival structures that are fairly consistent with California architecture from the time (as opposed to the Colonial Revival structures, which are anomalous in the region).

- Make your way through Fort Winfield Scott and follow Ruckman Ave. past some housing. Bear left onto Ruckman Ave. toward the Highway 1 overpass, walk beneath the pass, and turn left on wide Lincoln Blvd. A little ways down, beyond the stables where equestrian park rangers are based, turn right on Cowles Ave. Turn left on McDowell Ave.

- Just beneath elevated Doyle Dr.—recognizable for its orange rails that reflect the style of the Golden Gate Bridge (which Doyle feeds into)—pay a visit to the folksy Pet Cemetery, where you can pay respects to well-loved critters named "Skippy," "Knucklehead," and "Peep, Pet Pigeon of Johnnie Burke." Take a look around. It's by turns touching, humorous, and overblown. You will also notice that trucks and materials for the ongoing construction work on Doyle Dr. has nearly, though not quite, overwhelmed the tiny cemetery.

- Across from the Pet Cemetery, turn right on Crissy Field Ave., which follows the shadow of Doyle Dr. to meandering Lincoln Blvd., which sweeps past the military cemetery on its way to the Main Post and Parade Ground. Sheridan Ave. is a shortcut to the southern end of the Parade Ground, so turn right on it. The grounds have been converted into a parking lot, which adds convenience but detracts from the beauty of the surrounding buildings. Turn right on Montgomery St., where the historic Colonial Revival structures, uniform in design, were once barracks housing for enlisted men.

- Turn left on Moraga Ave. and you'll reach the Officers' Club, which still has some adobe walls from the original commandant's headquarters, built in 1776. Other parts of the building were added throughout the 19th and 20th centuries, but go inside and enter the Mesa Lounge (to the left immediately after you enter), where a cutaway reveals some of the old adobe. Note the deep recesses in the walls for the windows— it's a thick old structure. The National Park Service keeps its information center within the Officers' Club, so drop in for maps and books.

● Head back along the east side of the Parade Ground, past the Walt Disney Family Museum, which chronicles Disney's life and career from Steamboat Willie to Tomorrowland with drawings, home movies, and innovative machinery. Continue to Lincoln Blvd. and follow the road down to the Letterman Digital Arts Center, where many branches of George Lucas' multimedia empire, including Industrial Light and Magic (Lucas' Oscar-winning special effects company), are based. Walk around Building B, where (to borrow a familiar dyslexic patois) a fountain presided over by a statue of Yoda is. After admiring the Yoda Fountain, walk through the buildings into the complex's parklike grounds. The grounds are certainly interesting but are far too carefully landscaped, with perfectly shaped mounds carpeted with an impeccable lawn. An artificial stream trickles down to a "lagoon." Walk through or around the gardens, depending on how enchanted you are, and head out via Gorgas Ave. Turn right on Halleck St., pass back under Doyle Dr., and cross over to Crissy Field. From here it's just about 100 yards back to where you started.

POINTS OF INTEREST

NPS Visitors Center **Moraga Ave., 415-561-5444**

Warming Hut **Crissy Field, 415-561-3040**

Walt Disney Family Museum **104 Montgomery St., 415-345-6800**

route summary

1. Start at the Crissy Field parking lot and follow the cinder trail toward the Golden Gate Bridge, all the way to the Warming Hut.

2. Past the Warming Hut, walk on the sidewalk along the bay to Fort Point.

3. From Fort Point, backtrack toward the Warming Hut, looking for a trail that heads uphill, across from the Warming Hut.

4. Follow the trail up to Battery East and beneath the bridge toll plaza all the way to the coastal overlook.

5. From the coastal overlook head inland, along Landon Ct.

6. Cross Lincoln Blvd. to Fort Winfield Scott.

7. Pass through Fort Winfield Scott and look for Ruckman Ave. on the other side.

8. Follow Ruckman Ave. to Lincoln Blvd. and turn left.

9. Turn right on Cowles St.

10. Across from the Pet Cemetery, turn right on Crissy Field Ave.

11. Bear right onto Lincoln Blvd.

12. Bear right onto Sheridan Ave.

13. At the Parade Ground turn right on Montgomery St.

14. Turn left on Moraga Ave.

15. Turn left on Graham St.

16. Turn right on Lincoln Blvd.

17. Bear left on Letterman Dr.

18. Enter the Letterman Digital Arts Center through the passage next to Building B (past the Yoda Fountain).

19. Past the grounds and "lagoon" of the Letterman Complex, turn left on Gorgas Ave.

20. Turn right on Halleck St. and walk beneath elevated Doyle Dr. back to Crissy Field.

The Warming Hut at Crissy Field

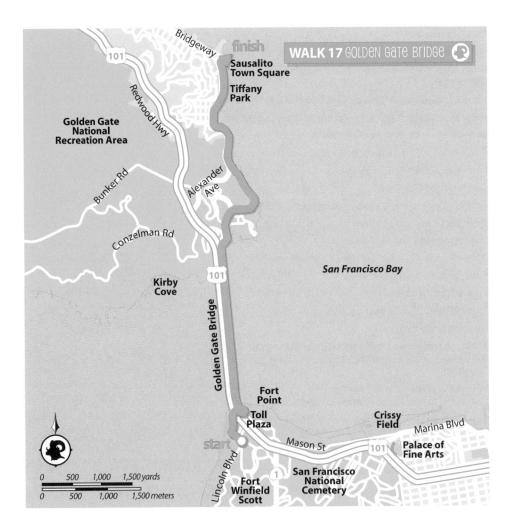

finish

Sausalito
Town Square

Tiffany
Park

Bridgeway

101

Redwood Hwy

Golden Gate
National
Recreation Area

Bunker Rd

Alexander
Ave

Conzelman Rd

101

Kirby
Cove

San Francisco Bay

Golden Gate Bridge

Fort
Point

Toll
Plaza

Crissy
Field

Marina Blvd

start

Lincoln Blvd

Mason St

101

Palace of
Fine Arts

Fort
Winfield
Scott

1

San Francisco
National
Cemetery

0   500   1,000   1,500 yards

0   500   1,000   1,500 meters

17 GOLDEN GATE BRIDGE: SPANNING TURBULENT WATERS WITH GRACE

BOUNDARIES: **From Fort Winfield Scott in the Presidio to the Sausalito Ferry Landing**
DISTANCE: **Approx. 4 miles**
DIFFICULTY: **Easy (but exercise caution walking the shoulder of the road into Sausalito)**
PARKING: **Public Transit is recommended for this walk. However, there are spaces on Lincoln Blvd., opposite the softball field near Fort Winfield Scott**
PUBLIC TRANSIT: **28, Muni bus; Golden Gate Transit buses following Marin County–San Francisco routes, San Francisco–Sausalito ferry, which docks at Pier 39 at Fisherman's Wharf.**

People who have never been to San Francisco or know very little about the city, at least know about the Golden Gate Bridge. The taut swag of its cables, recognizable in silhouette form, are an emblem of the city. Its color, International Orange, is associated specifically with the bridge. The bridge stands apart from the city—buffered by the parklands of the Presidio on the south end and the Marin Headlands on the north end—and its structure and natural setting complement one another. Very subtly, however, the bridge gets the upper hand over its environs. The bridge is obviously not as old as the hills that receive either of its ends, but the hills nevertheless appear to be there for the bridge. And the fog, which has always poured into San Francisco Bay through the Golden Gate strait, seems to serve the purpose of dramatically enhancing the bridge, concealing and unveiling its two towers and continually adjusting the natural light reflected on the bridge during the day. Ultimately, of course, the bridge serves us, making it possible for human traffic to travel to and from Marin County and beyond. Most thoughtfully, the bridge has a walkway on its eastern side so it is possible to cross the Golden Gate on foot to admire the views and ponder all that this bridge stands for. It was designed as a monument to progress, and if we are awed by the bridge, we must be awed by ourselves.

This walk starts in San Francisco and ends at the ferry terminal in Sausalito, so plan accordingly. The ferry ride from Sausalito to Fisherman's Wharf is a perfect way to finish your outing, but if you have parked in the Presidio, you will need to continue from the ferry terminal by bus back to the parking area near the Golden Gate Bridge. The entire length of the bridge itself, including approaches, is 1.7 miles. This walk is more than twice that distance, so be ready for some exercise.

● Start near the corner of Lincoln Blvd. and Merchant Rd. Rather than head down Merchant Rd. toward the bridge toll plaza, walk toward the sea cliffs to inspect a collection of old military batteries, such as the Battery Boutelle, which hasn't been in use since World War I. From here the Golden Gate—the narrow mouth of the bay and the widening funnel of the sea cliffs that embraces the Pacific—comes fully into view. Since pedestrian traffic on the bridge is restricted to the walkway on the bay (east) side, this rugged strait on the ocean side is often overlooked. To fully appreciate this perspective, walk over to these army battlements and follow the unpaved trail that leads from here to the bridge. To the northwest is Point Bonita, punctuated by its lighthouse in the Marin Headlands. To the southwest, the Cliff House marks Point Lobos on San Francisco's coast. Very likely a container ship is passing between these points on its way to Far East ports and another nearly identical ship is issuing forth beneath the bridge, as part of the continual movement of cargo in and out of San Francisco Bay.

● The trail clings closely to the Presidio's ragged cliffs and through terrain that's currently undergoing dramatic transformation as the Golden Gate National Recreation Area clears out Army landfill and nonnative plants. It isn't pristine, but it doesn't lack appeal. Here and there the trail affords flattering vantage points of the bridge, including a much-photographed angle from which the distant north tower appears to fit snugly within the south tower.

● The path soon dips beneath the bridge's south viaduct for an up-close look at its trussed and riveted underside, a treat for anyone interested in the engineering details. The viaduct here extends over two concrete pylons flanking the top of Fort Point. An artful arch braces the two pylons, and hidden in the works you may notice the bridge cables slicing downward to their southern anchorage. All that concrete beneath the south viaduct houses the cable anchorage. Much thought went into the design of this structure to protect picturesque Fort Point, which dates back to the Civil War. (The fort saw no action, but during the war San Francisco Bay was considered vulnerable to Confederate attack.) You can spend an hour here simply marveling at the sheer enormity of what went into creating the Golden Gate Bridge—the mind-boggling quantity of materials and the ingenuity behind it all.

- After passing beneath the bridge, follow the trail that curves up to the south parking lot, where you'll soon be in the company of hundreds of tourists who have come from around the world to see the bridge and snap a few photos.

  Before making your way onto the bridge, look for the statue of Joseph Strauss, the chief engineer who guided the bridge's planning and construction. Strauss submitted his first plans for a bridge to span the Golden Gate in 1917. After several major revisions, and arguments with the War Department over the advisability of building a bridge above the mouth of an important harbor, Strauss settled on an all-suspension design and then oversaw its construction from January 1933 to May 1937. He did not work alone, of course. He hired structural engineer Charles Ellis and other advisors to help solve challenges posed by the span's length and the depth of the channel, as well as strong currents, stiff winds, and the possibility of earthquakes. He also brought on architects John Eberson and Irving F. Morrow, who contributed the bridge's elegant Art Deco style. Strauss commendably went to greater-than-usual lengths to protect the safety of the workers building the bridge. Some nineteen workers were saved by netting Strauss insisted on installing beneath the building sites; still, eleven men died during construction of the bridge. Strauss himself died, while recovering from exhaustion, just twelve months after the bridge opened.

  Also in the plaza overlooking the parking lot, look for the cross-cut section of cable, some 36 inches in diameter. It's a persuasive demonstration of the bridge's unseen power. Don't bother to count the thick wires bound together within the cable: there are 27,572 of them.

- Continue onto the bridge. As you walk, stay alert for cyclists. On crowded days, the mixed traffic gets awkward and, occasionally, tense. Looking down, you'll notice you are still above land for a while, and below the bridge you can see the roof of Fort Point. Once you've cleared Fort Point, you have reached the bridge's suspension span, and you will see the cable rise at an oblique angle toward the south tower.

- Pause at the south tower to inspect the bronze plaques acknowledging the bosses of the men who hoisted the cables and poured the concrete and risked their lives for this bridge. The tower is 746 feet tall, as is the north tower. Standing next to it, you will notice the tower is a sound barrier that offers respite from the bridge's constant thrum of traffic. Look up to appreciate the design of the tower. It is stepped: each segment is slightly narrower than the one beneath it, each braced by horizontal trusses that are masked by decorative plates embellished with a repeating chevron motif. Corbels beneath the trusses further contribute to the textured design of the towers. Of course the towers are hardly aesthetic in purpose. They support the bridge's two cables, each weighing some 160 tons, and the cables in turn support the suspension span. The bridge is literally being held up from above, its weight distributed along the entire length of its cables.

● The main span between the two towers is 4,200 feet long. Pause again at the point midway between the two towers and look down. The water beneath the bridge is where the Pacific Ocean and San Francisco Bay meet. The water here is never calm. It chops and eddies and looks somewhat menacing. You might spot a sea lion swimming with evident playfulness barely below the water's surface, and a few pelicans may coast on loping wings beneath the bridge. Sailboats, cruising vessels, tankers, and tugs frequently travel through the Gate's narrow channel, all reflecting the Bay's never-ending enterprise and sport. Nevertheless, death lurks in those waters. By now, you may have noticed the CHP officers on bikes, who stop to chat with anyone who looks lonely or desperate. ("Hey, how's your day going?" is the usual opener.) You have probably spotted the phones for crisis counseling (or the curious sign that says ANY PERSON WHO WILLFULLY DROPS OR THROWS AN OBJECT OR MISSILE FROM ANY TOLL BRIDGE IS GUILTY OF A MISDEMEANOR). You may as well face it: many people have jumped from the spot at which you now stand, and from spots all along the walkway between the two towers. The water below appears ever ready to receive the next broken victim, to suck him or her down to undercurrents that stream out to sea, where crabs and sharks await.

● Before you sink into a maudlin state of mind, keep walking, until you've reached terra firma once again. Continue beyond the end of the bridge, down the two-lane road to Sausalito. It's downhill the entire way, but there's no sidewalk, so stick to the shoulder and maneuver carefully around parked cars.

The affluent and picturesque town of Sausalito, formerly a fishing village, attracts hordes of daytrippers every day. Walking the waterfront, you may find a good spot for lunch, such as Poggio Trattoria, an untouristy spot near the Ferry Landing for pastas, wood-roasted meats, and panini. Or you can purchase a sandwich at Venice Gourmet, an aromatic delicatessen near the Ferry Landing, to eat on the boat ride back to San Francisco. The Ferry Landing is near Sausalito Town Square, at Anchor St. and Humboldt Ave. Check www.goldengateferry.org for current ferry schedules. Getting out on the water is the perfect complement to a bridge walk. The air is fresh and the continual surge of the water beneath the boat gives you a palpable sense of the powerful immensity of the bay and the graceful bridge that spans the Golden Gate.

POINTS OF INTEREST

Poggio Trattoria **777 Bridgeway, 415-332-7771**

Venice Gourmet **625 Bridgeway, 415-332-3544**

Sausalito Ferry Landing **Anchor St. and Humboldt Ave.**

ROUTE SUMMARY

1. Start in the Presidio, at the corner of Lincoln Blvd. and Merchant Rd., walking toward the sea cliffs.

2. Follow trail past old battlements, along cliffs, beneath the Golden Gate Bridge.

3. Emerging from beneath the bridge, where trail splits, continue to the right, up to the parking lot, and continue on sidewalk onto the bridge.

4. Cross the bridge to the Marin County side.

5. Follow the two-lane road about a mile to Sausalito, and stay on Bridgeway along the town's waterfront, to the Sausalito Ferry Landing.

The south tower

Union St

Green St

Green St

Buchanan St

Laguna St

Vallejo St

Vallejo St

Octavia St

Gough St

Broadway

Franklin St

Van Ness Ave

Broadway

Fillmore St

Pacific Ave

Jackson St

Jackson St

Washington St

Washington St

Webster St

Fillmore St

Clay St

Lafayette Park

Clay St

Alta Plaza

Clay St

Laguna St

Sacramento St

finish

start

California St

Steiner St

Orben Pl

Webster St

Buchanan St

Pine St

Octavia St

Pine St

Austin St

Gough St

Franklin St

Bush St

Wilmot St

| 0 | 100 | 200 | 300 yards |
| 0 | 100 | 200 | 300 meters |

18 Pacific Heights: Victorian Splendor

BOUNDARIES: **California St., Franklin St., Broadway, Fillmore St.**
DISTANCE: **2 miles**
DIFFICULTY: **Moderately strenuous**
PARKING: **Off-street parking is available at 1700 California St., just off Van Ness Ave.**
PUBLIC TRANSIT: **California St. cable car; 1, 47, 49 Muni buses**

San Francisco's elite moved up to Pacific Heights' lofty, rarified environs back in the 1870s and have never left. Well, the original people have died, but their latter-day ilk remain. It seems Nob Hill wasn't big enough for all of the incredibly wealthy citizens of the Victorian city, and the well-to-do staked their claim to hilltop lots here to complement their vast estates down in San Mateo County. The grandest mansions in the Heights were once (and in some cases are still) homes of magnates, tycoons, industrialists, and dignitaries who also have office towers, parks, and streets named for them. Contemporary millionaires from the film and entertainment industry have joined the club relatively recently. Thus, this tour is largely an appreciation of jaw-dropping architectural phenomena. Interestingly, the neighborhood is densely packed, with front and side yards as rare as in any other part of the city, and many streets are dominated by luxury apartment buildings. On a weekday morning, sightseers will share the sidewalk with dog walkers and stroller-pushing nannies.

● **Start at the corner of Van Ness Ave. and California St., historically a key intersection for the neighborhood. Here the California St. cable car line terminates, but in the 1870s this line and several others continued up from the downtown area to the top of Pacific Heights, making the area accessible to residents in pre-automobile days. The lines ran up and down most of the east-west streets of the neighborhood. Initially Van Ness Ave. was a residential street where some of the city's very wealthiest built their mansions. At 125 feet wide, Van Ness is the city's broadest thoroughfare. Ironically, during the 1906 conflagration the street's hoity manses were systematically dynamited to create the firebreak that stopped the flames from climbing farther west. Van Ness was rebuilt as a retail strip, and by the middle of the 20th century was lined with steakhouses and flashy auto showrooms.**

● Head one block west on California St. and you'll begin to see what remains of the neighborhood's Victorian grandeur. The mansion at 1701 Franklin St. was built by Edward Coleman, a '49 gold miner who, unlike most, actually struck it rich. It stands on a large corner lot, which is typical for Pacific Heights—the biggest houses stand on corners, the smaller ones mid-block. Up near the eves the house is banded by a whimsical ornamental trim, with a recurring motif of laurels and torches. The Franklin St. side has a comely stained-glass window.

● Turn right (north) on Franklin. Another stately corner mansion stands at the intersection of Franklin and Clay. Now occupied by the Golden Gate Spiritualist Church, this white wedding-cake house was built for the Crocker family in 1900. The church meetings that go on inside are much more interesting. Founded in 1924 by Rev. Florence S. Becker, the congregation practices the Spiritualist rite of communing with the dead. Among the church's beliefs is that "the existence and personal identity of the individual continue after the change called death." Services are conducted by mediums. A little farther on the same side of Franklin St., actor Nicolas Cage owned the large Victorian at No. 1945 for many years.

On the next block of Franklin St., at No. 2007, the Haas-Lilienthal House cuts an impressive figure. Built in 1886 for William Haas, the austere house is one of the city's finest Victorians and reflects the elegance that once typified the neighborhood. Haas' daughter, Alice Haas Lilienthal, lived in the house until 1972, and it was turned over to the Foundation for San Francisco's Architectural Heritage a year later. It's open for tours several days a week ($10).

● Turn left at Jackson St. and left again at Octavia St. This curved, cobbled block was designed to slow traffic as it passed the immense Spreckels mansion, at the top end of the block. Adolf Spreckels, son of sugar magnate Claus Spreckels, built the grand chateau in 1925. Today, romance novelist Danielle Steele lives in it, and she evidently favors the vital decay aesthetic, for the mansion's exterior is faded and peeling. The house appeared as the nightclub Chez Joey in the 1957 film *Pal Joey,* starring Frank Sinatra, Kim Novak, and Rita Hayworth.

Lafayette Park, across from the Spreckels mansion, is little more than an overgrown hilltop with windblown patches of lawn where dogs sniff at each other. The park's leveled peak was the sight of Samuel Holladay's mansion during the latter half of the 19th century. Holladay was a prominent citizen—he was a judge who also served on the city council—but there was no record of his ever having purchased the land here. The city regarded him as a well-to-do squatter and tried to evict him, but Holladay knew the ins and outs of the law well enough to evade the city's efforts. He lived here until his death in 1915, and the city demolished the house in 1930.

● Turn right at Washington, and you'll quickly reach the gates of the Phelan mansion, at No. 2150. It was the home of James Phelan, who served as the city's mayor from 1897 to 1902 and in the U.S. Senate from 1915 to 1921. The Renaissance revival structure is awkward, with an unusual glassed-in mezzanine over the front entry. The former mayor's greatest architectural legacy is the Phelan Building, on Market St. (see the Lower Market St. walk).

● Turn right at Laguna St. A block up, the corner house at 2090 Jackson is the Whittier mansion. Just prior to the U.S.'s entry into World War II, this honey-toned sandstone house was purchased by the Nazi government, which intended to use it as a consulate. Those plans were obviously waylaid by the war.

● Continue on Laguna and turn left at Broadway. A block and a half up, the huge house at No. 2120 is one of two Flood mansions on the street. This one, built in 1901, was the home of Jennie Flood. It was built by her brother, James Leary Flood, who was the son of silver king James Clair Flood. Jennie was living in her father's Nob Hill mansion, which was damaged in the 1906 quake, so she moved here. James Leary Flood left a few years later, after building a new home up the street, at No. 2222, for himself and his wife. The second Flood estate, consisting of a nearly identical pair of massive villas, was completed in 1915. It is now the outrageously posh home of the Sacred Heart School, a Catholic academy.

● Having just passed Webster St., double back and turn right (south). The house at 2550 Webster is the Bourn mansion, a dark brick fortress with fantastic chimneys. It was built in 1896 for William Bowers Bourne, inheritor of the Empire Gold Mine, the richest mine in the state. The house was not Bourn's home—just a luxurious pit stop for entertaining guests while he was in town. Willis Polk was the architect.

● Turn right at Pacific Ave. and turn left onto Fillmore St., the principal commercial street of Pacific Heights. It's lined with clothing boutiques, beauty salons, restaurants, and cafes. Nice places to stop for dinner are Jackson Fillmore, an intimate little Italian spot, and the Elite Cafe, an exquisite old-town noshery offering an oyster bar and a decent Cajun menu.

● Turn left at California St. The corner of California and Webster is dominated by the magnificent Temple Sherith Israel, one of the pillars of the city's well-established Jewish community. The congregation dates back to the 1850s, and this awesome temple went up in 1904. It is more spectacular inside than out, with a frescoed inner dome and beautiful stained-glass windows conducting a brilliant spectrum on sunny days. Albert Pissis was the architect.

● Three blocks down, at 1990 California, the Atherton House looks humble, considering the size of the Atherton family's fortune. Faxton Atherton owned a huge estate that spanned the Peninsula south of San Francisco. The exclusive city of Atherton is named for him. After his death, his widow built this house for her frequent social calls to the city. It was built in 1881.

● From the Atherton House, it's just a few blocks back to Van Ness Ave.

POINTS OF INTEREST

Haas-Lilienthal House 2007 Franklin St., 415-441-3004

Jackson Fillmore 2506 Fillmore St., 415-346-5288

Elite Cafe 2049 Fillmore St., 415-346-8668

route summary

1. Start at the corner of Van Ness Ave. and California St.
2. Head west on California St.
3. Turn right on Franklin St.
4. Turn left on Jackson St.
5. Turn left on Octavia St.
6. Turn right on Washington St.
7. Turn right on Laguna St.
8. Turn left on Broadway.
9. Pass Webster St., then double back and turn south on Webster St.
10. Turn right on Pacific Ave.
11. Turn left on Fillmore St.
12. Turn left on California St.

Haas-Lilienthal House

Montgomery St

California St

Pine St

Bush St

Market St

Montgomery St

EMBARCADERO start

Justin Herman Plaza

Rincon Park

MONTGOMERY ST

Mission St

Main St

Beale St

Fremont St

1st St

Spear St

Bay Bridge

80

Mission St

Minna St

Natoma St

Howard St

Tehama St

Harrison St

Bryant St

Embarcadero

Yerba Buena Gardens

Hawthorne St

Folsom St

Essex St

2nd St

Delancey St

San Francisco Bay

Moscone Center

3rd St

Rizal St

80

Folsom St

Shipley St

Clara St

5th St

Bryant St

Welsh St

Ritch St

Zoe St

Freelon St

3rd St

Park Ave

Brannan St

2nd St

4th St

Townsend St

King St

Berry St

AT&T Park

finish

Terry Francois St

0   200   400   600 yards

0   200   400   600 meters

19 EMBARCADERO (SOUTH): THE DOCKS OF THE BAY AND A BASEBALL BONUS

BOUNDARIES: **Mission St., Spear St., Embarcadero South, King St.**
DISTANCE: **1¾ miles**
DIFFICULTY: **Easy**
PARKING: **There is off-street parking at 50 Howard St. Street parking is all metered and limited to two hours.**
PUBLIC TRANSIT: **Embarcadero BART station; F streetcars (street level); J, K, L, M, N, S streetcars (underground); 1, 2, 7 14, 21, 71 Muni buses**

In recent years, no part of San Francisco has changed as much as the waterfront south of Market St. The development of luxury condominiums, high-rise office towers, and the Giants' ballpark AT&T Park has brought new life to an area long ago abandoned by the shipping industry, which moved across the bay to Oakland in the late 1950s. Public art adds color and interest, as do restaurants and bars that get lively before and after baseball games, which is a good time to take this walk. (See the Sporting Green in the *San Francisco Chronicle* for a schedule.) Here and there are remnants of the Embarcadero's long-gone stevedore days. On this tour we'll take a close look at the ongoing development of this precious strip of real estate and hopefully catch a few innings of baseball free of charge.

● Start at the Rincon Annex Post Office, on the corner of Mission and Spear streets. It's no longer functioning as a post office, and as you can see from the street the modern Rincon Center rises up over the building's backside. The historic post office is an Art Deco beauty, dating to 1939, that has been preserved in near pristine condition and now serves as a unique foyer to the office tower. It was saved from demolition in 1978 primarily to protect the murals that grace the interior. Step inside for a look. From 1946 to 1948, Russian-born Anton Refregier painted 27 scenes depicting California history. Some common threads address concerns about freedom of speech and worship, for as Refregier worked on the murals such liberties were threatened in Europe, where Communism was spreading, and also in America, where anti-Communist paranoia had its grip on the country. Refregier's unromanticized scenes are populated by serious, often somber characters. Pass through the lobby into the newer Rincon Center and you'll reach a large, classy food court, with tables and chairs arranged around a "rain column"—water pours from the ceiling, several floors above, expands as it falls, and then appears to collapse neatly as it hits a stone platform on the floor. Your best choice for a light bite here is Yank Sing, one of the best dim sum restaurants in the city.

● A block east down Mission St., at Steuart St., the Audiffred Building looks like no other San Francisco landmark. It was built in 1889 by Hippolyte d'Audiffred, a French immigrant who in San Francisco sold charcoal to Chinese laundries and parlayed his earnings into real estate. He is believed to have designed this building himself, although he had no training as an architect. Consequently, the Audiffred building is an unusual amalgam of styles—a New England–style brick structure, with Victorian and Gothic details, capped with a mansard roof reminiscent of d'Audiffred's native France. The ground floor was originally occupied by the Bulkhead Saloon, popular with sailors and wharf hands, and the Coast Seamen's Union kept offices upstairs. Local legend maintains the building survived the 1906 fires thanks to a savvy barkeep, who bribed the fire department with a cart of wine and whiskey. The surrounding buildings all burned to the ground while drunk firemen trained their hoses on the Audiffred Building. During the early 1950s, the upper floors served as artist lofts, and poet Lawrence Ferlinghetti (who also paints) was among the creative souls who rented space here. Today, the ground floor is occupied by Chef Nancy Oakes' excellent Boulevard Restaurant, and its interior design is redolent with Belle Epoque details. The restaurant jumps during the weekday lunch hour, when free-spending office workers pour into its swank booths, and its bar is always a lively spot for a classy cocktail.

Across Mission St. is a monument to the striking longshoremen who were gunned down by police during a demonstration in 1934. It was on this corner that police fired into the crowd, killing Howard Sperry and Nick Bordoies.

● Continue around the Audiffred Building and turn right onto the Embarcadero. No. 250 is headquarters for the Gap company, well-known purveyors of casual clothing. The company was founded in 1969 by Donald and Doris Fisher and has grown to include more than 3,000 stores. The Gap began by marketing inexpensive blue jeans for teenagers. (The name refers to the "generation gap.") Peer through the building's glass doors for a look at Richard Serra's huge metal sculpture, which dominates a five-story atrium. It's called Charlie Brown, although it bears no resemblance to Charles M. Schultz's prematurely bald cartoon character.

● Cross the Embarcadero at Folsom St. for an up-close look at *Cupid's Span,* sculptor Coosje van Bruggen's 60-foot-high representation of the little cherub's bow and arrow, looking as though it fell from the sky and embedded itself into the ground here.

● Continue walking along this side of the Embarcadero. By now, you're already enjoying a wonderful perspective of the Bay Bridge, which you'll soon be walking under. On the way, at Harrison St., you'll pass the Hills Bros. Coffee Building, with its huge, eye-catching neon sign, and Gordon Biersch, a brew pub. Just as you reach the shadow of the bridge, take note of the fire station at Pier 22½, where two antique fireboats are docked. *Phoenix,* which was built in 1954, was used to pump water out of the bay to douse fires in the Marina after the 1989 earthquake. Afterward, Marina residents donated funds to purchase *Guardian,* a lovely vessel built in 1951.

The underbelly of the Bay Bridge is an awesome sight. The size of the bridge, and the effort that went into building it, are difficult to comprehend, especially from this informed vantage point. The bridge hits land at the southern side of Rincon Hill, which in the 1850s and '60s was the city's most fashionable neighborhood. It was here that the first millionaires of the Gold Rush city built their magnificent mansions. There's no sign of the hill's former splendor, as the area declined following development of Nob Hill in the 1870s. After more than a century of neglect, compounded by construction of the bridge in the 1930s, new condominiums and offices, including the 60-story One Rincon Hill, are going up in this part of town, making Rincon Hill once again a desirable address.

● On down the Embarcadero, at Pier 28, you'll spot an old tavern left from the waterfront's heyday. Called the Hi Dive, it's a smart little joint where you

Willie McCovey statue swingin' for McCovey Cove

might enjoy a beer and a view of the bay. At Pier 30, in an unprepossessing little shack suspended over the water is Red's Java House, a classic once patronized by old salts and longshoremen. It still attracts average Joes today, along with suited office workers. Head on in to this historic joint. In back, toward the loo, the walls are covered with photos by Bruce Steinberg, taken in 1971. These include shots of Red himself, looking every bit the wiry and fierce-tempered grill chef. He doubtless ran an orderly establishment. Red is no longer around, but you can still order a greasy cheeseburger and a cold bottle of Bud for a mere $6.

- Immediately to the south is a dead zone of parking lots. Pier 36 is slated for demolition to make way for a new waterfront park that, in its development stage, is being billed as the Brannan Street Wharf. The schedule is for a 2014 completion.

- Moseying on down the waterfront, keep your eyes peeled for the historical marker at the far end of Pier 30, which lists the names of 23 men who died while building the Bay Bridge.

- The ballpark begins to exert its gravitational pull here, especially before games, when a stream of pedestrians will be headed in that direction. Approach along the bay, through South Beach Harbor, where sailboats and yachts are docked. The huge Coke bottle and antique mitt loom over the left-field bleachers. Follow the curve of the stadium, to where the right field arcade overlooks McCovey Cove. Along this side of the ballpark an iron gate permits a view to nonpaying fans, who are allowed to stand here and watch part of a game from the field level, just a few paces beyond the right field warning track. Staff clear the area every three innings to make room for a fresh crowd. Every few months or so one of the ballplayers launches a titanic home run that plops into McCovey Cove, and it's usually a race between kayakers and dogs to see who can retrieve the ball.

- Walking in the same direction around the ballpark leads to a statue of Juan Marichal, the legendary Dominican pitcher whose menacing, high-kick delivery was a beautiful sight to Giants fans. Marichal pitched for the Giants from 1960 to 1973. A little ways farther is Willie Mays Plaza, with a statue of the greatest ballplayer to wear a Giants uniform. Some say he was the best, period. For two decades Mays hit for power, stole bases, and played the outfield with extraordinary ability, intuition, and spirit. Mays began his career with the New York Giants in 1951, coming to San Francisco when the team relocated in 1958.

● At Willie Mays Plaza, turn left onto 3rd St. and cross the Lefty O'Doul Bridge, named for Francis "Lefty" O'Doul, a ballplayer who won the National League batting crown in 1929 with a remarkable .398 average. San Francisco was his hometown. O'Doul managed the San Francisco Seals, of the Pacific Coast League, from 1935 to 1951. The bridge named for him is a charmer, a Strauss trunnion bascule span built in 1933 that crosses narrow Mission Creek.

● Once you've crossed the bridge hook left and walk along McCovey Cove on the opposite side from the ballpark. This is China Basin Park. You'll reach a statue of Willie McCovey, the slugging first baseman who was known as "Stretch" for his great size and for his ability to reach for wild throws to first. McCovey began his career in 1959 and retired in 1980. Also in the park is a perfect T-ball field, with a pint-sized diamond for pip-squeak ballplayers.

POINTS OF INTEREST

Yank Sing 101 Spear St., 415-957-9300

Boulevard Restaurant Mission St., 415-543-6084

Hi Dive Pier 28½, 415-977-0170

Red's Java House Pier 30, 415-777-5626

AT&T Park 24 Willie Mays Plaza (corner Third and King), 415-972-1800

route summary

1. Start at Rincon Center (the former U.S. Post Office), corner of Mission and Spear streets.

2. Walk east down Mission St toward the bay.

3. Turn right onto the Embarcadero.

4. Walk down to Folsom St. and cross the Embarcadero.

5. Continue down Embarcadero, beneath and then past the Bay Bridge.

6. Follow walkway along the bay front as it veers away from street, along South Beach Harbor.

7. Continue to the ballpark, then around it, along McCovey Cove.

8. At Willie Mays Plaza, on 3rd St., turn left and cross Lefty O'Doul Bridge.

9. On the other side of the bridge, turn left into China Basin Park.

Cupid's Span

California St

Market St

Montgomery St

Kearny St

Mission St

Minna St

Howard St

Folsom St

Geary St

Yerba Buena Ln

New Montgomery St

O'Farrell St

2nd St

Harrison St

San Francisco
Museum of
Modern Art

Mint
Plaza

Turk St

The
Warfield

80

Mint St

South
Park

start

4th St

San Francisco
Bay

Mary St

finish

Market St

5th St

3rd St

Mission St

AT&T
Park

Howard St

6th St

Bryant St

The Embarcadero

Folsom St

Harrison St

Brannan St

8th St

4th St

3rd St

9th St

7th St

80

280

0   300   600   900 yards

0   300   600   900 meters

10th St

144

20 SOMA: SLOUCHING SOUTH OF THE SLOT

BOUNDARIES: **Market St., 4th St., 2nd St., Natoma St.**
DISTANCE: **1½ miles**
DIFFICULTY: **Easy**
PARKING: **5th and Mission garage**
PUBLIC TRANSIT: **Powell St. BART station; 30, 45 Muni buses; Market St. buses and streetcars**

South of Market has been in a state of metamorphosis for decades. The area around Yerba Buena Gardens, once a grid of skid rows, is now firmly established as a zone of conventions and culture. Moscone Center and the San Francisco Museum of Modern Art (or SFMoMA) anchor the district. Farther to the west by just a few blocks, however, traces of the neighborhood's down-at-heels past remain. Taking it all in makes for an interesting study in contrasts as the transformation of SOMA continues apace.

● Start at Donut World on the corner of 6th and Market streets and stroll south on 6th St. for one block. As skid rows go it is somewhat tame, but you will see many run-down shops and cheap eateries in the mix: a taquería, a Louisiana Fried Chicken outlet, liquor stores, and loan shops. A couple of nightclubs on the block are dead during the day and flash to life around midnight. Tu Lan Vietnamese restaurant roils day and night with the energy of a steamship engine room. At the San Francisco Barber College you can get your hair cut by an apprentice barber for $8. And, most importantly, there is an abundance of residential hotels. Like the Tenderloin, on the other side of Market, 6th St. is home to the jobless and the would-be homeless. It is lively and colorful, though undeniably troubled. Many residents here suffer from poor mental health and substance-abuse problems, but overall this does not feel like a rock-bottom boulevard. More than thirty years ago, South of Market was block after block of similar housing for society's marginal characters, but as you will soon see, most of the old neighborhood is long gone.

● The intersection of 6th and Mission streets shows signs of transition, with an X-rated video superstore on one corner offset by Miss Saigon, a Vietnamese restaurant that looks classier than Tu Lan, and next to that a contemporary SOMA loft-style building.

However, if you gaze beyond Mission, it will be apparent that 6th St. doesn't change much in the blocks ahead. Turn left onto Mission and walk down a block that by comparison to 6th St. is quiet and also somewhat drab.

● Approaching 5th, you'll spot the home of the *San Francisco Chronicle*. The "Voice of the West" has occupied this building since 1924. By the paper's own account, it was founded in 1865 by brothers Charles and Michael de Young, who were teenagers at the time and in possession of a $20 gold piece, which they borrowed. The paper quickly established itself as a legitimate news source when it scooped the city's other dailies with the news of Lincoln's assassination. It was the city's only afternoon paper, and in the age of the telegraph the timing worked in the *Chron*'s favor. Like most newspapers today, the *Chronicle* is limping along with drastically reduced staff and dwindling advertising returns, and its future is a huge question mark.

● Turn left down Mint St., an alley behind the Old U.S. Mint. The sandstone Mint building is in good shape considering it was built in 1874 and has been empty for years. The city recently handed the deed of the Mint to the San Francisco Museum and Historical Society, which hopes to open it to the public, with exhibits on the city's history, in the not-so-distant future.

● Mint St. leads to Jessie St., which along the Mint's left flank has been made into a public square, with a stone patio and orange plastic chairs strewn about for conversation or people-watching. A number of cafes and restaurants have opened around this plaza, and during the lunch hour outdoor tables are set up in the shadow of the Old Mint Building, bringing life to a once neglected alleyway. Blue Bottle Coffee, on the ground floor of the San Francisco Provident Loan Association building, is an impeccable laboratory of caffeinated geekdom where single-source coffees burble in siphon pots. Needless to say, San Francisco's obsession with caffeinated beverages ceaselessly reaches for new levels of intensity.

● The next block of Mission St. is defined by a block-long parking garage on one side and the sleek glass back of the Bloomingdale's department store on the other. At the end of the block a partial view opens up on the Yerba Buena Center, the result of a 30-year project to transform 87 acres of "dilapidated hotels" into a shopping, convention, and cultural district.

More than a century ago, South of Market was known as "South of the Slot," for the cable car slot that ran down Market St. It was home to immigrant families and to migrant workers, a considerable proportion whom were seasonal laborers who mined the foothills and cleared Sierra forests. While between jobs or during the winter, they meandered back to the city, where they flooded into South of Market's bounty of residential hotels. It was a domain of bachelors. When Gold Rush-era fires and the 1906 quake destroyed parts of San Francisco, South of Market itinerants came in handy for the rebuilding effort. More often, though, they were forced to stretch meager savings over fruitless winters. They ate cheap meals in diners and found their entertainment in pool halls and theaters. Free lunches could be had in saloons and at rescue missions. Many had a propensity to drink and went broke before the arrival of spring. Able-bodied men were often reduced to panhandling. The injured and aged had little hope of ever seeing a paycheck again. The Great Depression broke many a man's back here, and the neighborhood declined and never recovered. By the mid-'60s, South of Market, like the Tenderloin to the north, was a grid of skid rows, its residents largely subsisting on monthly relief checks. The city's Redevelopment Agency fixed its eye on the area. They met with resistance from tenant groups, but in the end the agency had its way, sweetening the deal with museums and the promise of cash trickling down from conventions at Moscone Center. Demolition of block after block began in the late 1970s and, along with President Ronald Reagan's policy of slashing federal aid to urban programs, coincided with a dramatic jump in the city's homeless population.

● Continue east on Mission St. Cross 4th St. and continue a few steps down Mission to Yerba Buena Lane on your left, a pedestrian route that cuts directly to Market St. The walkway links the San Francisco Marriott Hotel, the Contemporary Jewish Museum, and St. Patrick's Church. The gleaming tower of the Marriott is a much-reviled piece of architecture. It is commonly likened to a jukebox, but San Franciscans would probably appreciate it if it looked more like a jukebox and less like a hotel. The Contemporary Jewish Museum occupies a historic power substation, with modifications designed by architect Daniel Libeskind, who found time to draw these plans while winning the contract for the new World Trade Center towers in New York. The power substation façade, designed by Willis Polk in 1907, survives in its entirety, with Libeskind's off-kilter cubes, colored a somber shade of night blue, jutting above the roof and adjoining the west side of the building. The museum itself has galleries devoted to art, history, and ideas, all relating to the Jewish people. St. Patrick's

Church, originally the parish of Irish Catholics who lived South of the Slot, was built in 1872. A century ago, it was believed to have had the largest congregation west of Chicago. Enter the church for a look at the stained-glass windows. Some members of the predominantly Filipino congregation here may be lighting votive candles or crawling, in a display of humility, up the aisles toward the altar.

● On the other side of Mission St., the cool Metreon shopping center opened at the height of the dot-com frenzy. Hence the late '90s vibe. Many of the original shops, including showcases for Sony and PlayStation products, barely survived the '90s, and the place no longer seems like the wave of the future. On a quick wander through you'll find a videogame arcade that specializes in semi-classics from the 1980s. (Pac-Man, Donkey Kong, and Space Invaders are all conspicuously absent.) Many of the game consoles have price tags on them. For a mere $595, "Turkey Hunting USA" can be yours to take home. On the other hand, you can probably master the game with a few dollars worth of tokens. There's also a bookstore (Books! In this day and age!) that sells the smartly designed volumes published by Chronicle Books—it's a shop without walls which, like an airport duty-free shop, seems designed to ensnare unwary shoppers who drift in. The Metreon multiplex cinema remains busy, and the building's current owners are transforming it into a food-centric mall, which is heading in the opposite direction from the place's original idea. This new direction may prove to be the right one. The Island Earth Farmers' Market, which takes over the ground floor every day, includes a great variety of vendors selling fresh tamales, Afghan bolanis (flatbreads stuffed with spinach, potatoes, and other ingredients), Moroccan hummus, and organic fruits and produce.

● Walk through the Metreon and exit through doors on the east side, facing Yerba Buena Gardens. The park is essentially an undulating lawn and a few trees, but it's a lovely urban space enhanced by an attractive skyline. Wander over to the elegant Martin Luther King Jr. Memorial, where a series of waterfalls pounds rocks below and drowns out your thoughts. Walk behind the falls to fully experience this reflective monument. From May to October, on weekends and some weekdays, a stage is set up on the lawn for live music and dance performances. It ranges from puppeteers to opera singers and is free.

● The Yerba Buena Center for the Arts takes up the 3rd St. side of the park, with exhibit spaces and a performing arts center. Although YBCA's galleries are spacious and well lit, this is not your ivory tower sort of museum. It emphasizes the work of living artists in all media, mostly with a local angle. Admission is $7.

● Follow 3rd St. back to Mission St. and turn right. On the next block, between 3rd and New Montgomery, are three museums. First is the Museum of the African Diaspora (MoAD), which exhibits the work of African and African-descended artists (admission $10). Across the street is the California Historical Society, a vaunted organization that serves primarily as a research facility with a huge library and a collection of historic photos, maps, and artifacts. It plucks gems from its collections for display in the back gallery. Admission is $3.

● The highlight of this block of Mission St. is the Cartoon Art Museum. The collection includes original drawings and inkings by a wide range of cartoon and comic artists. Little Nemo and Alley Oop strips share wall space with works by Chuck Jones, Charles M. Schulz, R. Crumb, and even a few Manga artists. You'll spot cels from Disney films as well as adult-oriented underground comix. It's a unique museum that really belongs here in San Francisco. Schulz (creator of Charlie Brown) lived in Santa Rosa, north of the city, and helped get the museum started. Crumb and *Ghost World* creator Daniel Clowes and a host of others have lived in and around the city. Admission is $6.

● At New Montgomery turn right. The striking Art Deco high-rise at 140 New Montgomery (at the corner of Minna St.) is the Pacific Telephone & Telegraph Building. It was designed by Timothy Pflueger and James Miller and built in 1925. A striking symbol of the telecommunications age, it was San Francisco's tallest skyscraper for three years. The building has been vacant since 2007.

● Head west on Minna, back to 3rd St. and SFMoMA. Designed by Mario Botta, the museum moved to these new digs in 1995 after residing in the Civic Center for many decades. It's an exceedingly popular museum, and the recent addition of the vaunted Fisher Collection (left by the founders of the Gap chain clothing stores, Doris and Donald Fisher) adds real depth. In fact, in less than 15 years the museum had out-grown its space and has announced expansion plans. Its photography collection is excellent, and fine traveling exhibits regularly stop here. Caffe Museo, overlooking 3rd St., is a fashionable spot for lunching and people-watching. Admission to the museum is $15.

● Head south down 3rd St., which leads to the Caltrain station, the ballpark, through the industrial "Dogpatch" neighborhood and Bayview-Hunter's Point, nearly reaching the city limits around Candlestick Point. (This walk doesn't follow it the entire way.) It is traditionally thought of as South of Market's "Main Street," though for much of its history its busiest blocks, between Market St. and the train station, were lined with gambling joints, saloons, and hotels that housed railroad workers and other transients. It was rough and tumble and it had literary appeal. Will Stevens, a one-time reporter for the *Examiner,* made it the setting of a Runyunesque novel called *Three Street,* in which the characters had colorful names such as Windmill Willie, Bookie Lou, and Johnny from Outer Space. Jack Kerouac, while working as a brakeman for the Southern Pacific, resided in one of this street's flophouses, and in the short story "October in the Railroad Earth" he wrote about "poor grime-bemarked Third Street of lost bums."

● The Redevelopment Agency took care of all that, at least up to the elevated freeway, two long blocks up. Continue south on 3rd. Just past the freeway, HRD Coffee Shop, at 527 3rd, offers a glimpse of the street's unesteemed history. The joint's starchy interior warmth puffs out from the open doorway, a come-on to anyone walking past it. Here and there you'll spot the unadorned brick side of old hotels, some with painted signs advertising ROOMS. Most of these are now offices.

● Past Bryant St. turn left onto South Park, a secluded city block shaped like a racetrack. The street loops around a pleasant green, with a playground and plenty of lawn that attracts more dogs than children. The street is a mix of Victorian residences, converted warehouses, and contemporary lofts, which reveals much, but not all, of South Park's history. In the 1850s, an Englishman, George Gordon, developed the land here as an exclusive community in the style of a London square. Elegant homes were built, and Gold Rush millionaires moved in. South Park's heyday lasted little more than a decade, as the rest of the South of Market area spread out and the working poor closed in on this tony little haven. By the time Jack London was born around the corner from here, in 1876, South Park was the home of immigrants and longshoremen. The '06 quake and fire destroyed the block, and many of the apartments and warehouses built in the quake's aftermath remain. Among these are the Sherman-Clay & Co. piano warehouse near the southeast corner. In the 1970s and '80s the street began attracting artists and soon acquired a post-industrial caché. In the late

'90s South Park was considered the heart of San Francisco's "Multimedia Gulch," as dozens of start-up companies opened shop in the surrounding blocks. That all ended abruptly in the early 2000s, but this quiet enclave retains a lively and interesting feel. Caffè Centro, for panini and hot Italian plates, and the South Park Cafe, for French bistro fare with a California twist, are great spots in which to unwind at the conclusion of a South of Market walk.

POINTS OF INTEREST

Blue Bottle Coffee Co. 66 Mint St., 415-495-3394

Yerba Buena Center for the Arts 701 Mission St., 415-978-2787

Museum of the African Diaspora 685 Mission St., 415-358-7200 (closed Sunday– Tuesday)

California Historical Society 678 Mission St., 415-357-1848 (closed Sunday–Tuesday)

Cartoon Art Museum 655 Mission St., 415-227-8666 (closed Monday)

San Francisco Museum of Modern Art (SFMoMA) 151 Third St., 415-357-4000

Caffè Centro 102 South Park St., 415-882-1500

South Park Cafe 108 South Park St., 415-495-7275

route summary

1. Start at the corner of 6th St. and Market St. and head south on 6th St. Turn left on Mission
2. Turn left on Mint St.
3. Turn right on Jessie St.
4. Turn right on 5th St.
5. Turn left on Mission St.
6. Turn left onto Yerba Buena Lane, the pedestrian alley that leads to the Jewish Museum.
7. Walk through the grounds in front of the Jewish Museum, around St. Patrick's Church, back to Mission St.
8. In front of St. Patrick's Church, take the cross walk across Mission St., to the Metreon shopping center.
9. Enter the Metreon on the corner of 4th and Mission streets and exit into Yerba Buena Gardens.
10. Follow the footpaths through Yerba Buena Gardens to 3rd St.
11. Turn left onto 3rd St.
12. Turn right on Mission St.
13. Turn right on New Montgomery St.
14. Turn right on Minna St.
15. Head south on 3rd St.
16. Turn left onto South Park.

HRD Coffee Shop, remnant of old 3rd St.

Duboce Park

start

Castro St
Walter St
Sanchez St
Belcher St
Church St
Market St
Landers St
Dolores St
Guerrero St

14th St
Henry St
15th St
Beaver St

14th St

15th St

Julian Ave

16TH ST MISSION

16th St

Mission St
Van Ness Ave
Shotwell St

Flint St
States St
Market St
Pond St
Church St

17th St
Ford St Dorland St

17th St

18th St

Diamond St
Collingwood St
Castro St
Hartford St
Hancock St
18th St
19th St
Cumberland St

Dolores Park

Linda St
San Carlos St
Lexington St
Valencia St

18th St

19th St

20th St

19th St
Eureka St
20th St
Liberty St

20th St

21st St

21st St
Diamond St
Hill St
Noe St
22nd St
Alvarado St
23rd St

Sanchez St
Church St
Vicksburg St
Quane St
Dolores St
Hill St

finish

Fair Oaks St
Guerrero St
San Jose Ave
22nd St
Bartlett St
Capp St
Van Ness Ave

24th St

24TH ST MISSION

Jersey St

0   200   400   600 yards
0   200   400   600 meters

154

21 DOLORES STREET: HIGH-TONED SIDE OF THE MISSION

BOUNDARIES: **Market St., Valencia St., 24th St., Sanchez St.**
DISTANCE: **2½ miles**
DIFFICULTY: **Strenuous (uphill climbs)**
PARKING: **Street parking is limited to two hours except on Sunday. The Market and Noe Garage (261 Noe St.) is three blocks from the start of this tour. Do not park at the Safeway across the street, as it is monitored.**
PUBLIC TRANSIT: **F streetcar; J Church train; 22 Muni bus**

Dolores St. is luxuriant without being snooty, grand but not opulent. For some 2 miles, the street's palm-shaded medians follow a straight and gracefully undulating path along the eastern edge of the Mission District. A walk along it takes in Mission Dolores, the panoramic vistas from Dolores Park, and inviting tangents up and down some of San Francisco's finest rows of 19th-century houses. It skirts the fringes of the Castro and Noe Valley. Apart from the Mission itself, this tour is not hugely concerned with landmarks or history. It's just one of the most beautiful walks in the city. We won't faithfully walk every block of Dolores St., opting instead to venture into the roller-coaster blocks of the Liberty Hill District and the northern rim of Noe Valley.

● Start at the corner of Dolores and Market streets, where the *California Volunteers* statue appears to be poised to ward off an invading army. The statue is worth a moment's appreciation, for it was created by Douglas Tilden, one of the city's finest artists at the turn of the 20th century. Tilden is widely known locally for works with somewhat overt homoerotic appeal, but this one, so near the Castro, is far more restrained. It's very dramatic, though, with its cavalryman jabbing the air with his sword as his horse tramples a fallen soldier who helplessly tries to aim his gun.

● Walk down Dolores St. Once you're past the huge car dealership, the street begins to take on its elegant character. Most of the buildings on either side of the street are apartment buildings. The palms in the medians are a popular pit stop for wild parrots. (The flocks here do not mingle with the flocks that habituate Telegraph Hill and parks in the north half of the city.)

● At 16th St., the huge Mission Dolores Basilica rises into view, and behind it is the humble Mission itself. Mission Dolores, built of four-foot-thick adobe walls and a clay tile roof supported by wood beams, is the oldest building in San Francisco, having been completed by 1791. When the mission was founded in 1776 it originally stood about a block-and-a-half east of here, on the shore of Laguna de los Dolores, an inland waterway that was later filled in. The Spanish missionaries conscripted local Indians to do their building for them, more or less in exchange for saving their souls. The surrounding lands were farmed by Indians along with Spanish families, though the settlement remained very small. The much larger Basilica was built after the 1906 fires destroyed an earlier cathedral on the site. Pope John Paul II said mass here on September 17, 1987. By all means, pay the $5 admission and take a self-guided tour. Beside the Mission, the cemetery is a highlight, in part because it is the only non-military cemetery within the city limits. Most of the names are worn off the ancient headstones, but interred here is an intriguing mix of dignitaries, paupers, and ordinary Joes from the 18th and 19th centuries.

● Two blocks down Dolores St., Mission High School's bell towers are a nice complement to Mission Dolores. Built in the Mission Revival style, construction of the school was completed in 1924. Author Maya Angelou and rocker Carlos Santana are alums.

● Just off the corner of Dolores and 18th St., you can get in line for ice cream at the Bi-Rite Creamery, an exceedingly popular spot for take-out soft-serve ice cream and sorbet. The "scream" is organic, high-quality stuff and includes some exquisite and unique flavors. Try a scoop of balsamic strawberry, or honey lavender, or malted vanilla. For something more substantial (a sandwich or salad), try to grab a sidewalk table across the street at Dolores Park Café.

● For the next few blocks, Dolores Park slopes up from the western side of the street. It's an amphitheater-like bank of green, with tennis courts, a soccer pitch, a playground, and lawns that are very popular among dog walkers and sunbathers. Continue on the sidewalk for a block, then follow the asphalt walkway up through the park toward the statue of Miguel Hidalgo, liberator of Mexico in 1810 (which, of course, included California at the time). Beyond the Hidalgo statue, cross the pedestrian bridge, which clears the Muni J Church streetcar tracks, then make a left onto the sidewalk just below Church St. The corner of Church and 20th is the southwest corner of the park and one of the great lookout points in SF. The J Church train is a pleasure to ride (you might want to catch one at the end of this walk) for views like this, as well as for the curving course the tracks follow through the backyards of the neighborhood.

● Turn left on 20th St., following the southern edge of the park, then turn right on Dolores. A block down, turn left on Liberty St. The south side of the block is a fine row of historic houses, all very different in style and all in tip-top shape. At Guerrero St., turn right. On the corner of 21st St., the house at 900 Guerrero is a stunner built by John Daly, an exceedingly successful dairy farmer, in 1895. Daly owned a huge tract of land south of the city. Parts of Daly City, named for him, were developed on land that had been his farm. The house here is in excellent condition, although it is no longer a single-family home.

● Turn left on Hill St. On the north side of the block is an impeccable row of nearly identical Stick-style Victorians, all built in the 1870s and '80s. These were originally middle-class homes.

● Turn left on Valencia and left again on 21st St., which we'll follow past Dolores St. up to Church St. At Church turn right, then turn left on Liberty St. It's a steady climb to the top. Stay on the north side of the street, where you can see the gardens that appear to be thriving along the median—hopefully, the sight of plants will make the uphill trudge easier to bear. At the top of the block, take the steps leading to Sanchez St. and turn left.

Mission Dolores

● A block up, the corner house at 3690 21st St. is a gingerbread cottage straight out of a classic Disney feature. It's called Casa Ciele ("sky house" in Spanish), which ought to feel appropriate enough if you're suffering from altitude sickness after hiking up to this point.

● It's all downhill from here, in a purely topographical sense. Follow Sanchez several blocks to 24th St., where you turn left to reach Noe Valley's main drag. The neighborhood is an enclave of millionaire couples, each raising one kid, and the street mostly serves local needs. You might have a good cup of coffee or spoil yourself by purchasing a new pair of designer shoes. If it's dinner time, backtrack to the corner of Douglass St., where Firefly serves up deservedly celebrated New American cuisine. To get back to where we started, walk down to Church St. and hop on a J train for a scenic ride.

POINTS OF INTEREST

Mission Dolores **3321 16th St., 415-621-8203**

Bi-Rite Creamery **3692 18th St., 415-626-5600**

Dolores Park Cafe **501 Dolores St., 415-621-2936**

Firefly Restaurant **4288 24th St., 415-821-7652**

route summary

1. Start at the Market St. end of Dolores St. and head south, to 16th St. and Mission Dolores.
2. Midway through Dolores Park, turn right up the asphalt path which leads to Church St.
3. Turn left at Church St.
4. Turn left at 20th St.
5. Turn right at Dolores St.
6. Turn left at Liberty St.
7. Turn right at Guerrero St.
8. Turn left at Hill St.
9. Turn left at Valencia St.
10. Turn left at 21st St.
11. Turn right at Church St.
12. Turn left at Liberty St.
13. Turn left at Sanchez St.
14. Turn left at 24th St.

Victorian beauty, Liberty Hill District

15th St

Valencia St

start Adair St

16th St

16TH ST MISSION

Camp St

Clarion Alley

Dearborn St

Sycamore St

18th St

Capp St

Van Ness Ave

Mission St

17th St

Shotwell St

Folsom St

Treat Ave

18th St

Alabama St

Bryant St

Mariposa St

18th St

Utah St

0   200   400   600 yards
0   200   400   600 meters

Lapidge St

Linda St

Guerrero St

Valencia St

San Carlos St

Lexington St

19th St

19th St

19th St

101

Liberty St

20th St

Harrison St

20th St

York St

Hampshire St

Capp St

21st St

Harrison St

21st St

Guerrero St

Ames St

Fair Oaks St

Hill St

22nd St

Mission St

22nd St

Folsom St

Treat Ave

Harrison St

Alabama St

Florida St

22nd St

Potrero Ave

San Jose Ave

Bartlett St

23rd St

24TH ST MISSION

24th St

Osage St

Lilac St

Poplar St

Lucky St

Balmy St

24th St

finish

25th St

22 THE INNER MISSION: TAQUERÍAS AND TATTOO'D BUILDINGS

BOUNDARIES: **16th St., Dolores St., 25th St., York St.**
DISTANCE: **2¼ miles**
DIFFICULTY: **Easy**
PARKING: **Off-street parking is available on the corner of Valencia and 18th streets.**
PUBLIC TRANSIT: **16th St. and 24th St. BART stations; 14 Muni bus**

San Francisco's most vibrant, diverse, and creative neighborhood is the Mission. The broad, flat district is populated by Latino families, artists, hipsters, and a growing number of white-collar workers. Amid the bars, bodegas, taquerías, and upscale restaurants are many buildings distinguished not so much by the businesses operating there, but by the art on the exterior walls. Murals—some in the tradition of Diego Rivera, others drawing on contemporary pop culture—are ubiquitous throughout the Mission. There are far too many works of art to take in on a single walk. This walk passes many of the key murals and ducks into a few shops to get a feel for the neighborhood.

● **Start at the corner of Mission and 16th streets, which is convenient if you're arriving on a BART train. Unfortunately, this busy intersection often feels like the end of the line for a growing number of junkies and prostitutes. But thanks to the station, there is plenty of foot traffic and the neighborhood isn't dragged down for long. Walk a block east on 16th and you'll reach the Redstone Building, at No. 2926. This building, also called the "Temple of Labor," is a meeting hall for labor unions. During business hours, enter to view the murals that cover every inch of wall in the lobby and hallways. The murals, including works by Barry McGee, Rigo, Aaron Noble, John Fadeff, and Sebastiana Pastor, were unveiled in 1997. Many of the works here echo the styles of the Depression-era artists who contributed pro-labor murals in Coit Tower and elsewhere in the city. The artists who worked on the Redstone Building are all associated with the Clarion Alley Mural Project (CAMP), and we'll see more of their works on the next stop of this tour.**

● Return to Mission St. and, after crossing, turn left on Mission and right onto narrow Clarion Alley. Without its continuous murals, Clarion Alley would just be a gritty alley inviting illicit activities. The alley's transformation began in the early 1990s, when artists living in an artists' loft midway up the block formed CAMP. The original group included Rigo, Aaron Noble, and Vince Oresman, among others, and some of their early works still survive on the alley's continuous wall of backyard fences and garage doors. Many other artists have joined them since. (Rigo and Noble have moved on, and the warehouse they worked in has since been demolished.)

The murals here on Clarion reflect the influence of pop art, comic books, outsider art, and graffiti. Critics sometimes categorize the Clarion painters, along with other Mission District artists, as the Mission School. Sometimes their diverse styles are lumped into a catch-all description: "urban rustic." Near Mission St., a work by Brian Tripp, a Native American artist, represents just one of many cross-cultural connections established by the Clarion Alley painters. The Mission Mural movement began as predominantly Latin American, with an obvious concern for immigration issues and the Reagan-era wars in Central America. Here the concept has broadened to embrace a post-punk and hip hop street aesthetic. A lot of the work, such as Matso's mural of ghosts emerging from the downtown skyline, are both political and cartoony. Clarion is a permanent work in progress. Over the years, weather has faded some of the older murals, while fresh new murals are continually introduced. Of late, taggers have had a hand in modifying the murals—Julie Murray's realistic elevator painting, midway up the block, is almost completely obscured. (Not surprisingly, Murray has also painted movie sets for a living.) More murals can be found one block north along Sycamore St.

● At Valencia St. turn right and then turn left at 17th St. Make a left at Dearborn St. As you approach 18th St. the spectacular Women's Building comes into view. The mural, called *Maestrapeace,* wraps like vines around two sides of the building. It was painted in 1994 by seven women artists, and thematically the painting celebrates women of all cultures. Walk a little ways up Lapidge St. to see the artwork on the building's east side.

● Return to 18th St. and turn right. The building on the corner of 18th and Lexington streets (on the Lex side) is covered with one of the neighborhood's more intriguing works. It's called *Generator,* and the artists are Andrew Schoultz and Aaron Noble. It's a finely crafted and unusual work, with cross-hatch shading and images of strange,

BaCKSTOrY: KINKY STUFF

In December 2006, a historic building in the Mission District was sold. The building is the old San Francisco Armory, a huge pile occupying an entire city block at 1800 Mission St., which was designed to resemble a Moorish castle. The buyer, Kink.com, is a producer of bondage films. So, just when people were starting to worry that the Mission was getting less interesting, along came the porn industry to the rescue.

Kink has used the site as a production studio for its fetish films, and the building appears strikingly well suited to the purpose. It has a menacing, Medieval exterior, and the last surviving stretch of Mission Creek runs through its dungeonlike basement. According to filmmaker James Mogul, the boiler room was tailor-made for a film set.

Kink has also hosted art festivals, open to the public and suitable for all ages, so occasionally it is possible to see what the building's interior is like without consenting to appear in a movie. Kink ownership has also entertained the idea of developing condominiums in the building, but with a catch: each unit would come equipped with cameras that could capture the residents' private moments on film.

intertwined birdhouses lurching skyward. It looks like something Dr. Seuss might have conjured up in one of his more harrowing tales. Note the way the artists incorporated the building's ventilation pipes and the power lines that cross in front of the painting. It's fun, intricate, and thought-provoking.

Follow Lexington to 19th St. and turn left. Turn right onto Mission St., one of San Francisco's liveliest and most interesting streets. Amid the taquerías and tiendas you'll see signs of the street's pre-Latino past, from a time when this was a largely Irish neighborhood. Some blocks are dominated by the faded and rusted beacons of grand old movie palaces that closed down decades ago. To get a real feel for the street, have a veggie burrito at Taquería Can-Cun (between 18th and 19th streets) or a carnitas taco at La Taquería (between 24th and 25th streets). Also, between 21st and 22nd streets, duck into Mission Market, a smorgasbord of spices, salsas, and produce for the Mexican-American kitchen. The market opens up into a small indoor

mall, where tables are set up in the middle and food stalls sell plate lunches and ras-
pados. On a busy day, it has the spirit and atmosphere of a market in Mexico.

At 23rd St. the side of a corner market has been covered with blank plywood.
Beneath the plywood a controversial mural has been preserved, despite having been
vandalized by someone who disagreed with the mural's political overtones, which are
sympathetic to the Palestinian cause. Being public, murals are naturally vulnerable,
not just to the natural elements but also to self-anointed cultural police. In this case,
the art has been saved by the plywood, but essentially is censored.

● Turn left at 23rd St. A few doors down, a barber shop is completely covered by *La
Lucha Continua/The Struggle Continues,* a mural comprised of portraits of political
and multicultural icons such as Pancho Villa, Martin Luther King Jr., Madame Nguyen
Thi Binh, Gandhi, Sitting Bull, and Che Guevara. The mural was directed by Susan
Greene, but was a collaborative effort (as are many murals) that resulted in a rich
variety of styles in the portraits. This is a "talking mural." If you are carrying a smart
cell phone, you can hear recordings about each subject by going to www.freedom
archives.org and clicking on *La Lucha Continua* in the left margin and then selecting
the names of the mural's subjects that interest you.

● Return to Mission and turn left. Continue on for a block and turn left onto shady
24th St., lined with shops, restaurants, and cantinas almost all catering to the Latin
American community. A few blocks down, turn right onto Balmy Alley, the Mecca of
the Mission District's mural arts scene. It's your classic back alley lined with garage
doors and backyard fences, but the entire length of it is covered with colorful murals.
Balmy predates Clarion Alley by nearly two decades. Some of the oldest murals on
the block were painted in the 1970s by Ray Patlán and a group of women artists who
called themselves Las Mujeres Muralistas—painters who favored the Mexican folk
styles that inspired Diego Rivera and José Clemente Orozco. At the time, their col-
lectivist politics, florid color schemes, and phantasmagoric compositions also would
have meshed fairly easily with the psychedelia of the Haight and the idealism of hippie communes. The machine guns are more Latin revolutionary than flower power,
however. Entering the alley from 24th St., Susan Cervantes' mural of a woman
dropping a baby from her private parts is sure to grab your attention, followed
by older murals inspired by Aztecan imagery and a mural depicting *campesinas*

wielding AK-47s. New murals appear all the time. Some of the more contemporary works are by artists cut from the Clarion Alley cloth, and while not apolitical, these are stylistically less tied to the traditions of the Latin American left. Some works make use of stencils, while others are inspired by cinema and comics. Toward the end of the block, a mural pays homage to classic Mexican film stars, including the comedian Cantinflas, painted by Rigo. Rigo, a native of Portugal, is one of the city's better known contemporary artists, having made a visible impact South of Market with prominent murals such as *One Tree* and *Inner City Home*. Here, in a more collaborative spirit, his work blends with the work of others. His Cantinflas shares the spotlight with an alluring dancing woman, painted by Carolyn Castaño. Walk to the end of the block and double back, taking in the art along both sides of the alley, and continue east down 24th St.

● Half a block down, at No. 2981, is the Precita Eyes Art Store and Visitors Center, which is a great place for learning about the local mural arts scene. Founded in 1977 by muralist Susan Cervantes, Precita Eyes has overseen many important commissions throughout the neighborhood, including along Balmy Alley, and the center's educational wing has produced many of the Mission's artists. The shop sells postcard photos of murals and T-shirts with murals on them. Anyone wishing to delve deeper into the culture can gather books and information here. Precita Eyes also organizes walking tours of the neighborhood's public art, sometimes led by local muralists.

● Across the street, past Alabama St., are a couple of very traditional Latino markets. Casa Lucas, at No. 2934, is a colorful shop that's useful if you're in need of a piñata or a bottle of guava juice. On the corner of Florida St., at No. 2884, La Palma Mexicatessen is a classic little purveyor of over-the-counter snacks, including excellent tamales and tacos. Grab a pack of hand-patted corn tortillas for an authentic treat. Sometimes you can spot women making them in the back of the shop.

● At the corner of 24th and Bryant streets, Galería de la Raza is a neighborhood institution that was founded in 1970 by artists involved in the Chicano civil rights movement. The gallery is an interdisciplinary space where art is exhibited and performances are staged. The gallery often showcases provocative and controversial art that usually casts perspective on topical issues such as illegal immigration.

● A block down 24th St. at York St., we can end our tour over a milk shake at St. Francis Fountain, a classic old ice cream shop that hasn't bothered to maintain museum-quality decor but is more comfortable for it. It's more film noir than Smithsonian. You can also get a burger or B.L.T. if you haven't already filled up on Mexican food.

POINTS OF INTEREST

Redstone Building 2926 16th St.

Women's Building 3543 18th St., 415-431-1180

Mission Market Fish & Poultry 2590 Mission St., 415-282-3331

Taquería Can-Cun 2288 Mission St., 415-252-9560

La Taquería 2889 Mission St., 415-285-7117

Precita Eyes Art Store & Visitors Center 2981 24th St., 415-285-2287

Casa Lucas Market 2934 24th St., 415-593-0785

La Palma Mexica-tessen 2884 24th St., 415-647-1500

Galería de la Raza 2857 24th St., 415-826-8009

St. Francis Fountain 2801 24th St., 415-826-4200

route summary

1. Start at the corner of Mission and 16th streets.
2. Head east on 16th St., cross Capp St., and enter the Redstone Building.
3. Return via 16th St. to Mission St., cross Mission St., and turn left.
4. Turn left on Clarion Alley.
5. Turn right on Valencia St.
6. Turn left on 17th St.
7. Turn left on Dearborn St.
8. Turn left on 18th St.
9. Turn right on Mission St.
10. Turn left on 23rd to barber shop.
11. Return to Mission St. and turn left.
12. Turn left on 24th St.
13. Turn right on Balmy Alley, walk a block up and back, returning to 24th St.
14. Continue on 24th St. and end at York St.

Balmy Alley mural

start

Duboce Ave

Erie St

101

14th St

WALK 23 MISSION Bars

Mission St

Van Ness Ave

Folsom St

Alameda St

Florida St

Bryant St

Ramona Ave

15th St

Capp St

16th St

Treat Ave

16th St

Franklin Square

Albion St

Guerrero St

Valencia St

Wiese St

Hoff St

16TH ST MISSION

17th St

17th St

Dolores St

17th St

Dorland St

Capp St

Shotwell St

Folsom St

18th St

Harrison St

Alabama St

Florida St

Mariposa St

18th St

Hampshire St

18th St

Lapidge St

Linda St

San Carlos St

Lexington St

Mission St

19th St

19th St

Dolores Park

Cumberland St

20th St

20th St

20th St

Liberty St

Guerrero St

Dolores St

Fair Oaks St

21st St

Hill St

Valencia St

Bartlett St

Van Ness Ave

Shotwell St

21st St

Treat Ave

Alabama St

Florida St

Bryant St

York St

finish

22nd St

| 0 | 200 | 400 | 600 yards |
| 0 | 200 | 400 | 600 meters |

23 MISSION Bars: HaPPY HOUrs, HaPPY FeeT

BOUNDARIES: **Duboce St., Valencia St., Folsom St., 22nd St.**
DISTANCE: **2¼ miles**
DIFFICULTY: **Easy**
PARKING: **Street parking can be difficult to find day or night. There is off-street parking at the corner of 18th and Valencia streets.**
PUBLIC TRANSIT: **16th St. BART station; F streetcar**

As the sun goes down on the Mission District, the neighborhood's vibrant murals fade into the shadows and irresistible artificial light splashes out onto sidewalks from the barrooms. This is one of the city's very best nightlife zones. The entertainment options are varied and of high quality, with a healthy mix of dives, supper clubs, and live-music venues. This tour selects several scattered spots, and you'll no doubt want to whittle it down a little further to avoid ending up in a gutter somewheres. A lot of ground is covered, and some of the streets are a bit dodgy at night. Use good sense while walking down dark blocks. You might also want to break a cardinal rule of walking tours and call on a taxi to bridge the gaps now and then.

● A fine place to start is Zeitgeist, where bikers and tattooed punk rockers hang out, on the corner of Valencia St. and Duboce Ave. The draw here, really, is the outdoor beer garden, which is nothing more than a graveled lot with picnic tables and a freeway ramp looming above it. Somehow, in the twilight on a warmish evening, this is one of the best places to be in San Francisco. You needn't be a local, a biker, or tattooed to feel at home here. You can grab a greasy burger and similar fare from a window next to the pool table.

● Before you get too comfortable out in Zeitgeist's backyard, head down Valencia St. several blocks to the Elbo Room, between 17th and 18th streets. The bar has been operating in some capacity or other since the end of Prohibition, but it has been a Mission District hipster magnet since the early '90s. If you can snare a stool at the sexy, curvaceous bar then you deserve a suave cocktail of some kind. When things get cranking here—9 or 10 p.m., usually—it can be difficult to get anywhere near a bartender or a server. Bands (rock, Latin, misc.) and DJs work the room upstairs. Have an early drink, return to 17th St., turn right, and mosey on.

● Next stop is the Uptown, at 17th and Capp streets. No part of San Francisco is known as Uptown, but why quibble over a name. This is one of the city's great dives. It doesn't look particularly welcoming from the outside (extra points for that) and the location couldn't be worse (more extra points), but step in and you'll have a hard time leaving. The old Formica booths and cool lighting are almost too perfect, but the place is real, very low-key, and more of a local than most of the hip Mission joints. Play some pinball or shoot some pool before moving on.

● A little farther down, on the desolate corner of 17th and Folsom streets, is the unas-suming Rite Spot Cafe. From the outside the bar appears to have been closed for years—it's a great look. Inside is about the same—slightly sleepy, slightly uncared for, slightly surreal. It's a supper club, with a long bar and a mess of tables and barely enough space for the band. The bands are of all stripes, and whoever books 'em is clearly bored with contemporary mainstream music. You can order Italian-American dishes—have the chicken cacciatore sandwich lathered in melted cheese and mayonnaise.

● From the Rite Spot follow 17th St. to Alabama St., turn right and continue to 20th St. The Atlas Cafe has been holding down this corner since 1996. The Atlas is a low-key, slightly arty coffee shop with an upbeat vibe. You can order beer, pizzas, and good sandwiches here. The only drawback is the place closes at 10 p.m. If it's a Thursday night around 8 p.m., definitely make this stop, since that's when the Atlas features live bluegrass music. On Saturday afternoons, from 4 to 6 p.m., it's ragtime.

● Continue on 20th St. to Mission St. The next couple of blocks have enough bars for a weekend bender. Just north on Mission, off 20th, you can't miss Bruno's bold, lit-up sign. It opened in the 1940s as a clubby Italian-American restaurant with sleek lines, mood lighting, and plush Naugahyde booths. In the '90s the place benefited from renewed interest in mid-20th-century swank and highball culture. An intimate jazz room was added. After a 2006 remodel, Bruno's is still a classy place for cocktails, but the musicians have been replaced by DJs.

● Turning around and heading south to the next block of Mission, between 20th and 21st streets, you come to Medjool, a relative newcomer, having opened in the 21st century. It's trendy and crowded, which can make it interesting and unpleasant at the same time. If the weather is nice, head up to the rooftop patio, where full bar service is available. In the downstairs lounge, you can order from a Mediterranean menu that covers the entire region's cuisine, from Southern Europe on around to North Africa.

● If you're still in a fashionable-contemporary mood, next door is Foreign Cinema, a one-stop shop for dinner and a movie. Just slip into the sultry Laszlo Bar for sophisticated concoctions and cool DJs after 9 p.m.

● Down the road a piece is another of the Mission's fine dives, Doc's Clock. Before entering, walk across the street for a good look at the sign, a real beauty that promises good times within. Past the seductively lit bar is a little room in which to drink and play shuffleboard. Doc's Clock often has interesting events planned, such as Doggie Happy Hour (bring along a pooch) and film screenings by local filmmakers. No cover.

● Turn right at 22nd St. The Make-Out Room, just off the corner, is a fine and idiosyncratic watering hole that's been a neighborhood stalwart for over a decade now. With an assemblage of Formica tables scattered over a concrete floor, it's nothing fancy, but the joint still has atmosphere and a certain amount of class. Many nights after 8 p.m. it features live bands—everything from cowpunk to indie rock—and charges a cover.

● If the music scene at the Make-Out doesn't steam your glasses, head up the block on 22nd St. to the Latin American Club, an equally unfussy yet appealing bar. These are distinctive and tranquil environs with a Mission-slacker bent—it's a good spot to settle into over conversation.

POINTS OF INTEREST

Zeitgeist **199 Valencia St., 415-255-7505**

Elbo Room **647 Valencia St., 415-552-7788**

Uptown **200 Capp St., 415-861-8231**

Rite Spot Cafe **2099 Folsom St., 415-552-6066**

Atlas Cafe **3049 20th St., 415-648-1047**

Bruno's **2389 Mission St., 415-643-5200**

Medjool **2522 Mission St., 415-550-9055**

Foreign Cinema **534 Mission St., 415-648-7600**

Doc's Clock **2575 Mission St., 415-824-3627**

Make-Out Room **3225 22nd St., 415-647-2888**

Latin American Club **3286 22nd St., 415-647-2732**

ROUTE SUMMARY

1. Start at Zeitgeist, corner of Valencia St. and Duboce Ave.
2. Head south on Valencia, past 17th St., and you'll reach the Elbo Room.
3. Turn right on 17th St. A block past Mission St., at Capp St., is the Uptown.
4. Continue on 17th St. At the corner of Folsom St. is the Rite Spot Cafe.
5. Continue on 17th St. to Alabama St. and turn right.
6. At 20th St. turn left. Just off the corner is the Atlas Cafe.
7. Turn around and follow 20th St. west.
8. Turn right at Mission St. Just off the corner is Bruno's.
9. Turn around and head south on Mission St. Just past 20th St. are Medjool and Laszlo.
10. Continue on Mission St. On the other side of the street, past 21st St., is Doc's Clock.
11. Turn right on 22nd St. Just off the corner is the Make-Out Room.
12. Continue on 22nd St. Near the corner of Valencia is the Latin American Club.

Doc's Clock

Cesar Chavez St

finish

start

Precita Ave

Precita Park

Bessie St

Precita Ave

27th St

Valencia St

San Jose Ave

Powers Ave

Mirabel Ave

Coso Ave

Shotwell St

Manchester St

Folsom St

Treat Ave

Harrison St

Alabama St

Tiffany Ave

Mission St

Fair Ave

Elsie St

Bonview St

Bernal Heights Blvd

Ripley St

29th St

Coleridge St

Lundys Ln

Prospect Ave

Winfield St

Bernal Heights Park

Bernal Heights Blvd

Carver St

Virginia Ave

Eugenia Ave

Kingston St

Bonview St

Bocana St

Chapman St

Powhattan Ave

Cortland Ave

Santa Marina St

Elsie St

Wool St

Andover St

Moultrie St

Anderson St

Ellsworth St

Gates St

Folsom St

Banks St

Eugenia Ave

Cortland Ave

Prentiss St

Nevada St

Nebraska St

Putnam St

Bronte St

0   100   200   300 yards
0   100   200   300 meters

24 Bernal Heights Park: a Dog's Fondest Dream

BOUNDARIES: **Precita Ave., Folsom St., Cortland Ave., Winfield St.**
DISTANCE: **2 miles**
DIFFICULTY: **Moderate (long uphill stretches)**
PARKING: **Street parking around Precita Park has no time restriction.**
PUBLIC TRANSIT: **24th St. BART station; 12, 14, 27 Muni buses**

Bernal Heights rises up from the southern edge of the Mission, where narrow streets dead-end long before they can reach this rocky, windswept hilltop. The broad views of the Mission, Potrero Hill, the bay, and the distant downtown skyline are fantastic—but that's par for the course in San Francisco. What makes this walk especially alluring is the suddenness with which the sheltered, slightly funky Bernal Heights neighborhood turns into a rugged chunk of wilderness. The hill is home to many red-tailed hawks that glide silently about the slopes looking for anything small that moves. Wear good hiking shoes for this one. And if you have a dog handy, bring it along and free it from its leash—you'll both fit right in.

● Start at Precita Park, in a pleasant residential pocket to the north of Bernal. You can grab a cup of coffee at one of the cafes on tree-lined Folsom St., which runs along the park's western edge. Turn left, heading south. Folsom rises steadfastly, as though developers entertained thoughts of making it clear the hill in a straight shot. However, within two blocks, as the going gets rough the road abruptly swerves to the left. Just as suddenly, you're above the rooftops, amid the grassy, rocky terrain for which Bernal Heights is known. If it's the rainy season, wind, clouds, and mist swirl about the green face of the hill. In spring, the hill is covered with wildflowers. In summer, its an arid scape of red rock and yellow grasses. There's a dog for just about every human up here.

● Folsom curves up to Bernal Heights Blvd. Turn right, pass the gate (which prohibits cars from entering), and you'll enter Bernal Heights Park. The road loops up a fairly easy incline around the hill. The long, straight boulevards that slice through the Mission District drop into view behind you. Down below the road, along the western side of the

BACK STORY: BERNAL HEIGHTS OUTDOOR CINEMA

Bernal Heights naturally attracts creative types, and to prove it, every fall the neighborhood showcases the works of local filmmakers in an outdoor film festival. Films are shown on Saturday nights during the months of September and October. The filmmakers usually give a talk in a local cafe, then everyone proceeds to a nearby park (sometimes Bernal Heights Park), where the film is shown as the sun goes down. It's a fun and social event.

Musician Michael Franti has shown his work in the festival, and Ralph Carney has scored films screened during the festival. The neighborhood's best known filmmaker is Terry Zweigoff, director of such delights as *Bad Santa* and *Ghost World*. So far, the festival hasn't featured Zweigoff's work. For information, check www.bhoutdoorcine.org.

hill, look out for narrow, unofficial trails (which at times fade beneath new grass or fallen pine needles)—these lead to hidden gardens planted by local residents on city property. The steps leading down to Esmerelda St. lead to some of these gardens.

- On the south side, where the road is gated, a wide, rocky path corkscrews up toward the top of the hill. The red rock here is chert, and is the same stuff found up on Corona Heights. Follow the trail up. On blustery days, you might see several hawks hovering in place about twenty feet overhead, their wings stretched wide, adjusting perceptibly to keep the wind beneath them. The birds keep very still up there, stealthily scanning the ground for potential prey. Stand beneath them and you'll have about as good a look (without the aid of binoculars) as you could ever hope to get of wild raptors in action.

- The path loops around the summit, with unbroken perspectives of the city and the bay. There are ledges and lookouts and little spur trails. It's not a huge area, but you'll want to roam about a bit before returning to Bernal Heights Blvd. A driveway leads down from the top. Look for Anderson St. and stroll on down past a hodgepodge of residential architectural styles. Bernal Heights was never a wealthy district, although today these homes sell for a pretty penny (as do all homes in SF). The narrow streets, many of which curve abruptly to avoid steep grades, give the area an off-beat, Montmartre-like feel.

● Follow Anderson down to Cortland Ave., the main commercial strip. Make a right; you'll find good places to eat, coffee shops, and a bookstore. Bernal doesn't generally draw much business from out-of-towners or even from people who live elsewhere in the city, making this a very neighborly sort of urban backwater. That's not to say it's backwards. Fine restaurants here include Moki's Sushi and Pacific Grill, for Polynesian, and the Liberty Cafe, where the chicken pot pie is legendary. Wild Side West is a funky lesbian bar that often draws a mixed crowd simply because it's the best watering hole on the hill.

● As Cortland begins to descend back down to Mission St. turn right on Elsie St. Just off the corner, note the 19th-century barn that was converted into a house ages ago. Two blocks down, Virginia curves up to meet Elsie. Follow it and you'll see some of the neighborhood's finest Victorian homes. Local residents are cultivating a garden along the right side of the road, beneath the curved retaining wall. A block down, turn right on Winfield St., which runs in a straight line to the north side of the hill. From here you can meander back to Precita Park, along the way discovering hidden pockets where the streets meet at odd angles. You have two straightforward choices: take a right on Coso Ave., which leads back to Folsom, or turn left on Coso and you'll soon reach pretty Mirabel Ave., which, if you turn right, gets you back to Precita Park.

Views from Bernal Hieghts

POINTS OF INTEREST

Moki's Sushi and Pacific Grill **615 Cortland Ave., 415-970-9336**

Liberty Cafe **10 Cortland Ave., 415-695-8777**

Wild Side West **424 Cortland Ave., 415-647-3099**

ROUTE SUMMARY

1. Begin at Precita Park and turn left up Folsom St.
2. Turn right onto Bernal Heights Park; enter the park.
3. Pass the gate onto the dirt road, making your way around the summit of the hill.
4. Turn left (south) on Anderson.
5. Turn right on Cortland Ave.
6. Turn right on Elsie St.
7. Turn left on Virginia St.
8. Turn right on Winfield St.
9. Take Coso right to Folsom St. or left to Mirabel Ave., either way returning to Precita Park.

View of the Mission District from Bernal Heights

Portola Dr

Turquoise Way

Duncan St

Diamond St

Castro St

Diamond Heights
Shopping
Center

O'Shaughnessy Blvd

Diamond Heights Blvd

rocks

Glen Canyon
Park

Marietta Dr

Teresita Blvd

preschool

rocks

Berkeley Way

Diamond St

Bella Vista Way

Arbor St

Diamond St

Sussex St

Elk St

Chenery St

Bosworth St

Glen Park
BART
station

start
finish

Mangels Ave

San Jose Ave

280

| 0 | 200 | 400 | 600 yards |
| 0 | 200 | 400 | 600 meters |

25 GLEN CANYON

BOUNDARIES: **Bosworth St., Diamond St., Portola Dr., O'Shaughnessy Blvd.**
DISTANCE: **2 miles**
DIFFICULTY: **Moderate (some hills, trails with loose rocks)**
PARKING: **Street parking on Chenery**
PUBLIC TRANSIT: **Glen Park BART station; 44, 52 Muni buses**

San Francisco's urban continuity is frequently broken by hills topped by outcrops of rock and mounds of soil yielding auburn grasses. In the case of Glen Canyon, the city gives way to a deep impression—a gash, really—where Islais Creek supports a rich riparian environment of arroyo willow, elderberry, blackberry, horsetail, monkeyflower, and eucalyptus. The canyon is filled with birdsong and the dull jackhammering of woodpeckers. Red-tailed hawks are likely to swoop overhead, a harmless snake may cross your path, and a coyote may blend into the scenery while sunning itself on the canyon's grassy slopes. A rare example of native coastal scrub survives along the park's western slope. Making liberal allowances for the nonnative plants and the hush of unseen traffic on O'Shaughnessy Blvd., a hiker in the rugged canyon might imagine San Francisco during the city's somnolent Californio days.

● Our walk begins and ends in the pleasant Glen Park neighborhood, where a picnic lunch can be assembled. The Glen Park BART station, if that's how you're traveling, is the most attractive station within the city limits, though it is by no means a landmark. From the station, at the corner of Diamond and Bosworth streets, follow Diamond St. through the intersection of Chenery St. to Sussex St. and turn left. Following Sussex uphill through charming residential blocks will get you to Diamond Heights Blvd. Turn right, continue uphill a little ways, and make a left onto Berkeley Way. Half a block farther, on the left side, a rocky outcrop signals an unsigned trailhead that descends into the canyon.

● Avoid the unstable ad hoc footpaths that head straight down the side of the hill and follow the main trail. It begins on the right side of the rocks and follows a gentle seam along the canyon's eastern wall. The trail passes through a small grove of eucalyptus, and then the earth becomes copper colored where chert has been ground into a fine soil. The entire extent of the canyon, less than a mile in length, comes into view. You'll see slopes covered with bunch grasses and oat grasses (green after sustained rains, golden brown in the summer), outcrops of crumbling chert, spreads of bramble, coyote brush and poison oak, and clumps of trees. Down among the rock crevices hides a rare and shy native, the San Francisco alligator lizard.

● The trail carves a wide arc down into the canyon floor, where a rocky outcrop is worth scaling. Along either side of the rocks, a couple of paths can be explored. One, to the north of the rocks, becomes a shaded path, completely closed in on either side by dense, low trees. This path ultimately rises to meet Portola Dr., so when you reach the end of the trees, turn back, pass the rocks, and look for the boardwalk that hems Islais Creek. Brooks such as this once ran throughout San Francisco, each one filled in or diverted through culverts as natural terrain was converted to cityscape. Islais Creek is a rare, though not unique, survivor. It is fed primarily by natural springs within the canyon itself.

● Past the boardwalk, the trail widens to accommodate service vehicles, and a nursery school appears in a dense eucalyptus grove to the right. The trail leads out of the canyon to some softball fields. Exit the park, turn right on Elk St. and left onto Chenery St., which leads back to the neighborhood's small shopping district. Here you can refortify yourself over a sturdy breakfast or lunch at Tygers, on the corner of Diamond and Chenery. Half a block up Diamond, Cafe Bello is a nice little coffeehouse.

POINTS OF INTEREST

Tyger's **2798 Diamond St., 415-239-406**
Cafe Bello **2885 Diamond St., 415-585-3457**

route summary

1. Start at the Glen Park BART station, on the corner of Diamond and Bosworth streets.
2. Head up Diamond St. and turn left onto Sussex St.
3. At Diamond Heights Blvd. turn right.
4. At Berkeley Way, turn left.
5. At the rocky outcrop, half a block up Berkeley Way, look for the unsigned trail heading down to the right.
6. Follow the trail along the eastern slope of the park, and where the trail curves below Portola Dr. turn left, down toward the rocks jutting from the canyon floor.
7. To the west of the rocks, follow the trail through the dense trees, and when you reach the end of the trees, turn back.
8. Having returned to the rocks, continue south on the trail, following it as it becomes a boardwalk alongside Islais Creek.
9. The trail meets an unpaved access rode, near the nursery school; continue on it until you reach the softball field.
10. Outside the park, turn right onto Elk St.
11. Turn left onto Chenery St. and follow it back to the Glen Park shopping district.

Rocky outcrops in Glen Canyon

start

McCoppin St

Otis St

Buchanan St

Market St

Pearl St

101

Scott St

Waller St

Hermann St

Duboce Ave

Clinton Park

Brosnan St

Duboce Park

Church St

Noe St

Walter St

Sanchez St

Belcher St

14th St

Dolores St

Ramona Ave

Guerrero St

14th St

Minna St

Alpine Ter

14th St

Henry St

Landers St

15th St

15th St

Julian Ave

Castro St

15th St

Beaver St

Sharon St

16th St

16TH ST MISSION

Hoff St

Market St

Prosper St

Pond St

Church St

Chula Ln

States St

17th St

Dorland St

Dearborn St

Lapidge St

Ford St

Dorland St

Dolores St

Guerrero St

Linda St

Valencia St

Lexington St

San Carlos St

Mission St

Hartford St

Noe St

18th St

18th St

Hancock St

Dolores Park

19th St

Church St

19th St

Eureka St

Diamond St

Collingwood St

Castro St

19th St

Cumberland St

Cumberland St

20th St

20th St

finish

20th St

Liberty St

Liberty St

0   200   400   600 yards

Liberty St

0   200   400   600 meters

26 Upper Market and The Castro: Gay Bars and Victorian Beauties

BOUNDARIES: **Market St., Octavia St., Douglass St., 20th St.**
DISTANCE: **1½ miles**
DIFFICULTY: **Easy**
PARKING: **You might try your luck along Guerrero or Valencia streets. Off-street parking is available at the Market and Noe Garage.**
PUBLIC TRANSIT: **F streetcar**

The Castro is probably the best known gay neighborhood in the U.S. Perhaps not coincidentally, it's also a treasure trove of lovingly maintained architectural gems, with unbroken strings of beautiful Victorian houses along many blocks. Formally called Eureka Valley, the neighborhood was home to a working-class immigrant community before gays began to drift out this way in the early 1970s. They were most likely drawn by well-priced Victorian houses and the winning location, with streets terracing up the eastern slope of Twin Peaks, which on most days shields the Castro from the fog. The neighborhood's quiet residential streets reflect the refined tastes of its denizens, who are by and large established professionals. Castro St. between Market and 18th streets is the busy commercial hub, with Upper Market taking on much of the spillover. This tour will take in both sides of the district: the elegant homes as well as the bars and clubs that reflect the Castro's social side. (The Twin Peaks walk explores the western part of the neighborhood, which climbs the western slopes of the prominent hills.)

● Over the years, the gay community has spread a ways down Market St., toward Civic Center, so we'll begin our tour well east of Castro St., at the corner of Market and Octavia streets. Here, at 1800 Market, The Center stands like a portal to the neighborhood. It offers services and programs for lesbians, gays, bisexuals, and transgenders, and also has a cafe. The Center is architecturally interesting, as it consists of a historic Victorian, painted a solid and sober blue that segues into a strikingly modern wing of tinted glass panels, which meet at oblique angles. It's a suitable introduction to the neighborhood, where an appreciation for the old does not reflect a fear of the new.

● Heading west on Market St., a few blocks up, on the same side of the street, you come to the Mint Karaoke Lounge, a little neighborhood dive that gets its name from the nearby U.S. Mint, which can be seen soon after you pass the bar. The Mint is a popular nightclub that draws a fairly mixed crowd, though it appeals mostly to hams eager for their turn at the mic. The U.S. Mint, up on the hill, is a foreboding structure that looks more like a futuristic military installation than a place that produced money. It no longer produces circulating currency but still churns out commemorative coins that are highly collectible. The Mint was built in 1937.

● Just below the U.S. Mint is a Safeway supermarket (at 2020 Market St.) that's more or less like any other Safeway except for its proximity to the Castro. People perusing the aisles in search of toothpaste or canned corn have noted that this place can be somewhat cruisy.

● Up Market St. a couple of blocks west, just before the corner of Sanchez St., is Cafe du Nord. The name is French, the architecture is Scandinavian, and the classy below-street-level joint is pure swank with a modern, hip edge. The onetime speakeasy is a mainstay on San Francisco's small-venue live music scene, with a regular lineup of independent acts, many local and mostly worth catching. Upstairs, the Swedish American Hall is no meatball parlor, but another excellent live music venue. It has the look and feel of a Masonic lodge, with heavy Alpine woodwork. Events are scheduled here infrequently, though.

● On the next block up, Lime is an interesting combination of eatery and nightclub. The gaudy decor could be straight out of a dream by the rock star Beck—a '70s vision of the future that grooves but isn't particularly appetizing. Naturally the joint jumps.

● Across Market St., at the corner of Noe St., Cafe Flore is a celebrated hangout where the patio tables are highly coveted on sunny days. As you can see, in construction it resembles a gardener's shed, though on a much larger scale. Potted greenery con-tributes to the effect. But Cafe Flore is about coffee, beer, light meals, seeing, and being seen. A block up is Catch, a well-regarded seafood restaurant.

● The corner of Market and Castro streets, where you turn left onto Castro, is naturally one of the principal crossroads of the neighborhood. A huge rainbow flag flaps in the wind from a pole high above Harvey Milk Plaza, at the southwest corner. Named for the assassinated city supervisor, the cramped little plaza is tucked between a building and the entry to the Muni station, but if your dogs are tired it offers a couple of benches.

- Across the street, Twin Peaks Tavern is known by younger people as "the coffin" because people under the age of 60 seldom drink in it. The bar is famous for its untinted picture windows, which were a novelty for a gay bar in the early '70s. The bar was open long before then, having served a blue-collar clientele for several decades.

- The neighborhood's biggest landmark is the Castro Theater, a few doors up Castro St. from the Twin Peaks Tavern. There aren't many movie palaces of this sort left, which is why the Castro is treasured by all San Franciscans. The programming is eclectic, featuring a mix of independent films as well as fine prints of the classics. Often, the movie is preceded by an artful performance on the house organ, and on occasion the Castro will screen silent films with a live pit orchestra. Several film festivals take place here. The building, a Moorish flight of fancy, is particularly dramatic at night, when the marquee is lit up. It was built in 1922 and the plans were drawn by architect Timothy Pflueger.

- A couple of doors farther along, Cliff's Variety is the neighborhood hardware store. It's been open since the 1940s. As with the Safeway, a common sort of store is made extraordinary by virtue of its location. Along with the usual plumbing and electrical fixtures, the store stocks plaster moldings for restoring 100-year-old houses and all the kitchen and bath supplies a happy homemaker might be looking for. It also has a fine selection of goofy toys of the sort that appeal to nostalgic adults. On the same block, A Different Light Bookstore is the city's leading gay-oriented bookstore. Several nights a week authors read from their works here.

- The bookshop is just a few paces from the corner of Castro and 18th streets, which is considered the nexus of the neighborhood. There are restaurants and hangouts in either direction along 18th St., but continue on Castro. At No. 575, Harvey Milk operated his camera store during the 1970s. Milk and his partner lived upstairs, and Milk conducted his campaign for supervisor here. A bronze plaque on the sidewalk commemorates his contributions to the local community.

● Just past 19th St., Castro St. turns residential, with an impressive row of Victorian apartment buildings stacking up along the incline. Turn left on Liberty St., which looks much as it would have over a century ago. Immaculate single-family homes, nearly uniform in character, line both sides. These were middle-class homes originally but are worth a pretty penny now.

POINTS OF INTEREST

The Center **1800 Market St., 415-865-5555**

Mint Karaoke Lounge **1942 Market St., 415-626-4726**

Cafe Du Nord **2170 Market St., 415-861-5016**

Lime **2247 Market St., 415-621-5256**

Cafe Flore **2298 Market St., 415-621-8579**

Twin Peaks Tavern **401 Castro St., 415-864-9470**

Castro Theater **429 Castro St., 415-621-6120**

Cliff's Variety Store **479 Castro St., 415-431-5365**

A Different Light Bookstore **489 Castro St., 415-431-0891**

ROUTE SUMMARY

1. Start at Market and Octavia streets and head west along Market St.
2. Turn left at Castro St.
3. Turn left at Liberty St.

Victorians on Liberty Street

Randall
Museum

finish

Castro
Theatre

start

17th St

Market St

18th St

Tankhill
Park

Corbett Ave

Caselli Ave

19th St

Douglass St

Collingsworth St

Castro Dr

Hartford St

Clarendon Ave

Kite Hill
Open Space

Seward St

Twin Peaks Blvd

Grand View
Terrace

Corwin St

20th St

Twin Peaks
Reservoir

Burnett Ave

Romain St

Market St

Eureka St

Diamond St

21st St

Gardendale Dr

Corbett Ave

Grand View Ave

22nd St

23rd St

Hoffman St

Elizabeth St

Twin Peaks Blvd

Hopkins St

Cole St

Belvedere St

Clayton St

0   200   400   600 yards

0   200   400   600 meters

27 TWIN PEAKS: SCALING THE MAGNIFICENT BUST

BOUNDARIES: **Market St., Danvers St., Corbett Ave., Twin Peaks Blvd.**
DISTANCE: **3 miles**
DIFFICULTY: **Strenuous**
PARKING: **Market and Noe Center, 2284 Market St., between 16th and Noe, has off-street parking.**
PUBLIC TRANSIT: **F streetcars (street level); K, L, M streetcars (underground); 22, 33, 37 Muni buses**

Twin Peaks has an allure that dates back at least to the Spanish years, when they were known as *Los Pechos de la Choca,* which is typically translated as The Breasts of the Maiden (or, sometimes, the Indian Girl). The current English name is more subtle but has become iconic to the point of overstatement. Both names make hay of the fact that these two hills, of comparable size, are paired off in a fairly precise arrangement. In fact, they are almost too perfect to be believed. Eighteenth-century Spanish Catholics might have attributed such a formation to the hand of God. A skeptic of today, however, might be more inclined to suspect unnatural augmentation. This walk requires some climbing on loose trails, so wear suitable shoes and expect to get some exercise.

● A walk up to Twin Peaks is an excuse to explore the Castro's back streets. Starting from the corner of Castro St., turn left and head west up Market St. on the south sidewalk. After several blocks, just after crossing Douglass St., turn down the pedestrian stairs onto Ord St., then turn right on 18th St. Another block up, Chan Chan is a friendly little hideaway that's good for Cuban sandwiches, ropa vieja, or a strong cup of Joe or even a mojito (though take our recommendation and save that for later—we have some strenuous hiking ahead). Across from Chan Chan, follow Danvers St. to Caselli, cross Caselli, and continue on the alley-like back street, which is still Danvers. At 19th St., turn left.

This part of the Castro may be San Francisco's most finely composed neighborhood. It has an ideal hillside setting and a solid collection of attractive, though not spectacular, Victorian residences. Eureka Valley, as the Castro is still often referred to, was long a working-class neighborhood with immigrants from Scandinavia, Ireland, and Germany. Some of these blocks are predominantly gay now, though recently gays have been dispersing into nearby cities and straight couples have been moving into the Castro. Architecturally, the neighborhood is consistent. Whereas the imposing estates of Pacific Heights were surrounded by large lots on which 20th-century apartment buildings would be built, the Castro's kit Victorians were put up, and remain, side-by-side, almost uninterrupted. The grid bends to the terrain here, giving the neighborhood a European feel while also making it possible to switchback up and down.

● Press on 19th to the corner of Yukon, where you will see Kite Hill, a scraggly open parkland with no apparent entrance. Continue a little way on the right side of 19th St. until you reach the first private garage, at which point a dirt trail should be plainly visible. Head up the trail, through gardens which rapidly yield to a wild, grassy mountaintop. Kite Hill seems a bit neglected, but it's more appealing for it. People live in San Francisco for decades without ever discovering this spot. For those who do make their way here, the views—of Castro rooftops and the downtown skyscrapers on one side, of a canyon-like neighborhood squeezed between Kite Hill and Twin Peaks on the other—are a big payoff. Regardless of the weather down below, it is very gusty on top, and one can instantly understand the name. A kite would surely soar high over the city from here. There's a bench, if all you want to do is sit and absorb the view.

● From the top of Kite Hill, look for the houses along a dead-end street immediately to the southwest. This is Grand View Terrace. Follow it down to Grand View St. and turn left. A few doors down Grand View Terrace, hidden between two houses, a hand-painted sign with a cartoon rooster on it shows the way down pedestrian-only Acme Alley. (If you can spot the hard-to-find addresses, look for numbers 61 and 65 Grand View, and you will see steps descending between them.) Walk carefully down the steps, as the risers are uneven, past half-hearted gardens and backyard fences, and take still more caution as the steps end, leaving you to negotiate a steep, loose-soil trail for the last 20 feet or so.

● Cross Corwin and enter a well-established community garden on the corner of Corwin and Acme Alley. These are dry gardens, well worth a lengthy pause to admire the impressive array of drought-resistant plants. Proceed downhill through the gardens, until you reach a small patio that is actually half of Seward Mini Park. Yes, the odd concrete structure you see before you is a pair of slides. They look as slick and curvaceous as an Olympic luge run and a little dangerous. Presumably these slides are for children, but no one would fault an adult for taking this quick route the rest of the way down to Seward St.

● At Seward, turn right, and stay on the elevated sidewalk, along the right side of the street. It's a beautiful block with lots of planting. At the end of the block, turn right onto Douglass. At 20th, Douglass hits an incline too steep for cars and the street turns into a concrete stairway for pedestrians. Walk up the steps, through another hillside garden, and at the top, continue along Douglass St., on the right-hand side through another well-planted block. By now, you might have come to the reasonable conclusion that this is San Francisco's Garden District.

● Turn right on Romain. Sutro Tower stands directly ahead, though it's still some distance off. Head two blocks up to Market St. This part of Market, an extension that dates to the 1920s, forms a rampart, cutting off the Castro from streets such as Corbett and Clayton, on Market's upside. The divide turned out to be advantageous for the Castro, making the neighborhood feel more sheltered and complete.

● Cross Market via the Romain St. pedestrian bridge, continue west up Romain, and make a left on Corbett St. After you pass Rooftop Alternative School, turn right at Hopkins St., and left onto Burnett Ave. Here the neighborhood takes an unexpectedly bland turn. It is evident that in the 1960s, Burnett Ave. and Gardenside Dr. were handed over to developers of very little imagination. Adjacent to the drab apartment complexes that proliferate here, concrete public stairways lead upward, and we'll take advantage of these now and follow a more scenic route back down. The steps lead all the way up to Parkridge Dr. where you turn right and which loops around and becomes Crestline Dr. A few paces from this hairpin curve in the road, you'll find a clearly marked trailhead to the right, with an arrow pointing up. Here a stepped unpaved trail leads us out of apartmentland, past low shrubs and brambles, up to Twin Peaks Blvd. and to the peaks themselves.

● It must be said, the peaks are a bit of a letdown when you first lay eyes on them from Twin Peaks Blvd. In fact, the boulevard, which forms a figure eight around the two peaks, is largely the problem. The road, paved in 1934, was carved like a too-tight training bra into the hills. The road also has unsightly waist-high concrete shoulder barriers, which may dissuade a dispirited walker from continuing all the way up to the peaks' blustery tops. But slide on over the barrier and forge upward.

● The views from the tops of both peaks are pretty special, and if you scale both hills, the effect is almost stereoscopic. From the south peak, Market St. appears as a prominent seam through the central city, leading the eye to downtown skyscrapers. Pan to the left for an attractive vantage of the Golden Gate Bridge and the Marin Headlands beyond. You can see the south peak's twin and, just behind it to the right, glimpse Alcatraz. Panning to the right along the bay you'll see Treasure Island and the Bay Bridge. South of Market St. are Potrero Hill, Bernal Hill, Candlestick Point, and the impressive San Bruno Mountain and, beyond that, the northern reaches of the Santa Cruz Mountains. To the west is Mount Davidson, San Francisco's highest peak, with its giant cross poking up above a surrounding grove of eucalyptus. On a cloudless day you can see the surf at Ocean Beach, which from this distance appears to break in supreme slow motion. On days of crystalline clarity, even the Farallon Islands, more than 25 miles away, can be spotted.

Looking immediately about you, the crumbling rock outcrops on which you stand obviously make a harsh habitat for plant life, but you'll notice ankle-high coast strawberries, blue wild rye, monkey flower, and yarrow. At times, pesky poison-oak shrubs run a bit wild until the Recreation & Parks Department cuts them back. If you brush against poison oak (be on the alert for the small, scalloped green leaves, turning reddish in summer) you can expect an unpleasant itch and rash. From up here it is often possible to look down on red-tailed hawks as they survey lower slopes for prey.

● Descend the south peak via the same trail you came up, cross Twin Peaks Blvd. and head up the north peak, where the view of downtown and the bay is closer, but also somewhat obstructed by radio towers immediately to the east. As you will notice, from this vantage the Ferry Building lines up perfectly at the foot of Market St. To the northwest, you'll have an unobstructed view of Sutro Tower, the giant three-pronged antenna that brought television to much of the city when it was completed in 1973. The awkward orange-and-white antenna still has its detractors, who were quick to object to its sci-fi implications back in the '70s, and it also has its fans, who are obviously unconvinced Twin Peaks would be prettier without it.

● The trail over the north peak continues down the other side. Follow Christmas Tree Point Rd., which might easily be taken as a third rung in the figure eight formed by Twin Peaks Blvd. Christmas Tree Point Rd. curves around the radio buildings, and along it is a popular vista that's accessible to motorists. There's parking and benches, and the view of downtown is excellent.

● At the end of Christmas Tree Point Rd. turn right on Twin Peaks Blvd. and follow it down. There's no sidewalk as the road hurtles downward, so be on your guard for cars. A sidewalk does materialize as the road becomes residential. You'll continue on Twin Peaks as it takes a sharp turn right at a small pocket park with a bench at Clarendon.

● At Graystone Terrace turn right and enter another picturesque hillside enclave. The lane crooks past Edwardian houses with Spanish revival details and finishes. Graystone crosses the Pemberton Steps, an attractive brick stairway that is flanked by hillside planting, including a number of young Japanese maples. Turn left and follow the steps down to Clayton.

● Cross Clayton St. and cut through the little rock and cactus garden fashioned with care from a triangular street corner. Turn left onto Corbett Ave. and follow it down to Danvers St., which leads back to Market St. and your starting point at Market and Castro.

POINTS OF INTEREST

Chan Chan Café Cubano **4690 18th St., 415-864-4199**

Sutro Tower, visible from the Castro

route summary

1. Begin at corner of Market and Castro streets and head west up Market, on the south sidewalk.

2. After crossing Douglass St. turn left, follow steps down to Ord St., which feeds directly to 18th St.

3. Turn right (east) on 18th St.

4. Turn left onto Danvers, cross at Caselli, and continue on Danvers (which now looks like a back alley).

5. Turn left on 19th St.

6. At Yukon, spot Kite Hill rising from the southeast corner, continue along the right side, past the gardens, and, immediately before the first garage, look for the trail, heading upward to the right.

7. Climb to the top of Kite Hill and look for Grand View Terrace, a residential cul-de-sac.

8. Follow Grand View Terrace to Grand View St. and turn right.

9. Turn left down pedestrian steps called Acme Alley (look for hand-painted sign).

10. At corner of Acme Alley and Corwin St., walk through community gardens, down toward Seward Mini Park, follow slide down to the bottom.

11. Turn right on Seward.

12. Turn right on Douglass.

13. At 20th, continue up the Douglass St. Steps.

14. At top of steps, continue on Douglass, along right-hand side, for one block.

15. Turn right on Romain St.

16. Take the pedestrian bridge at Romain, cross Market, and continue up Romain for one block.

17. Turn left on Corbett St., right on Hopkins St., and left on Burnett Ave.

18. About the length of a city block up Burnett Ave., steps to the right head uphill, through apartment buildings, all the way to Parkridge Dr.

19. Turn right on Parkridge Dr., follow its bend, where it becomes Crestline Dr., and continue about half a block to a marked trailhead on the right.

20. Follow the trail to the right, up the hill, to Twin Peaks Blvd. and climb over the low concrete barrier.

21. Cross Twin Peaks Blvd. and head up the trail to the top of the south peak.

22. Retrace steps down the south peak, cross Twin Peaks Blvd., and follow the trail up the north peak.

23. Continue over the north peak, down to the north loop of Twin Peaks Blvd. and, immediately north, follow the loop of Christmas Tree Point Rd.

24. Turn right at Twin Peaks Blvd. and walk down the shoulder. Continue on the sidewalk that eventually materializes around Burnett Ave.

25. Turn right at Graystone Terrace.

26. Turn left (down) on the Pemberton Steps.

27. Cross Clayton St., cut through the corner rock garden, and turn left on Corbett Ave.

28. Follow Corbett Ave. downhill to Danvers St. and turn right.

29. At Market St. turn left.

30. End at the corner of Market and Castro streets.

Turk Blvd

Golden Gate Ave

University of
San Francisco

Golden Gate Ave

McAllister St

Scott St

Pierce St

Steiner St

McAllister St

Fulton St

Fulton St

Grove St

Ivy St

Fulton St

finish

Alamo
Square

Hayes St

Baker St

Grove St

Webster St

Buchanan St

Lyon St

Hayes St

Fillmore St

Central Ave

Masonic Ave

Broderick St

Divisadero St

Fell St

Ashbury St

Oak St

Fell St

Panhandle

Page St

Page St

Steiner St

Oak St

Masonic Ave

Lyon St

Baker St

Page St

Pierce St

Laussat St

Ashbury St

Haight St

Scott St

Waller St

Central Ave

Germania St

Hermann St

Waller St

Buena Vista Park

Lloyd St

Duboce Park

Alpine Ter

Duboce Ave

Walter St

Sanchez St

Belcher St

Downey St

Delmar St

Buena Vista Ter

Noe St

Market St

14th St

Corona
Heights
Park

Castro St

Henry St

Church St

Landers St

Upper Ter

15th St

Museum Way

States St

Flint St

Beaver St

Clifford Ter

start

| 0 | 200 | 400 | 600 yards |
| 0 | 200 | 400 | 600 meters |

28 westside cordillera: corona Heights, Buena vista park, and alamo square

BOUNDARIES: **16th St., Central Ave., Golden Gate Ave., Steiner St.**
DISTANCE: **2½ miles**
DIFFICULTY: **Strenuous**
PARKING: **Two-hour street parking is available around Corona Heights, especially on 16th St. near the Flint St. entrance. Two hours doesn't leave enough time, so Sunday (when parking is unlimited) is a good day to make this walk. Off-street parking is available at the Market and Noe Garage.**
PUBLIC TRANSIT: **F streetcar; K, L, M Muni trains; 24 Muni bus**

The three hilltop parks in this tour are only a few blocks apart, but couldn't be more different. Corona Heights is a rocky outcrop just above the Castro District. Buena Vista Park's densely wooded terrain sprouts abruptly from the Haight. Alamo Square is a grassy quadrant amid classy Victorian houses. All have sweeping views of San Francisco, each offering a unique perspective, but the real pleasure of taking in all three in one shot is in passing through such varied topography within a short space. Wear good shoes for hiking and be prepared to traverse steep, unpaved trails.

● Assuming you've either parked your car or disembarked from public transit down in the Castro, start by climbing from the corner of 16th and Flint streets up to Corona Heights. From just about anywhere along upper Market St., if you look to the west, you'll see the red jagged cliff to which we're headed. You can reach park entrances by walking up 16th St. to Flint St. or by walking up Beaver St. above Castro St. Beyond the park entrances, most of the unmarked trails lead to the top, so walk on up. It's a pretty barren hill, with a few trees, grasses, and wildflowers.

● The most distinctive feature of Corona Heights is the rock itself. The reddish stone is visibly cracking up on the surface, and the trails are strewn with squared-off chips and chunks. Pick up a piece and look it over. This rock is chert, formed by plant and animal matter that settled on an ancient seafloor and became petrified before being thrust up here. Similar rock formations turn up elsewhere in the city, but Corona

Heights is the most striking example. The hill is crested by dramatic, jagged pin-nacles of rock, some of it spray painted on by taggers. From here, take a look around and enjoy a broad view of the city—in addition to the downtown skyline and City Hall, you'll see all of the South of Market area, the Mission, the Castro, Noe Valley, Twin Peaks, and, immediately to the north, Buena Vista Park (our next stop). At lower ele-vations of Corona Heights are a well-situated playground, the Randall Museum, and a patch of green where people can liberate their dogs from their leashes. The Randall Museum is an educational museum for kids that has a combined emphasis on nature and the arts.

● Descend the trail to the dog area and exit the park onto Roosevelt Way at Museum Way. Turn right on Roosevelt and bear left onto Park Hill Ave. A block up is Buena Vista Ave., which rings Buena Vista Park. Cross and turn left. The sidewalk here runs around the base of the park's southern slope. Opposite, the large peachy building at 351–355 Buena Vista Ave. East made a brief appearance in Hitchcock's *Vertigo*. Once you're past it, look for a narrow sandy path that heads up and follow it into the park's woodsy hillside. It leads to a maze of little spur trails, but try to stay with the widest available trail. This park has long been known as a gay cruising spot after dark. In the '60s, hippies frolicked here as well. Near the top, you'll reach an asphalt path that will serve you well the rest of the way. It winds to good lookout points along the north and east side of the park, and also dips down into a shady gulch that's very sheltered. By now you are surely appreciating the size and varied topography of this inner-city park. Buena Vista, originally called Hill Park, was set aside by the city as a park in 1867. Many of the trees were planted on behalf of Adolf Sutro, who annually observed Arbor Day by donating seedlings. John McLaren, who for half a century was superin-tendent of Golden Gate Park, also oversaw the forestation of Buena Vista Park.

● Find your way toward the western edge of the park. There's an exit near the end of Frederick St. Turn right onto Buena Vista Ave., which curves around the park and leads to Haight St. Along the way, take note of the mansion at No. 737. It was built in 1897 for Richard Spreckels, whose uncle was sugar magnate Claus Spreckels. In the house's early days, writers Ambrose Bierce and Jack London supposedly resided here briefly. More certainly, Graham Nash (whose surname fills this gap: Crosby, Stills, _____, and Young) lived here, as did actor Danny Glover for a time.

● Past Haight St., Yerba Buena Ave. becomes Central Ave. Follow it to the Panhandle, the strip of shady greenery between Oak and Fell streets. Cross the park to the Fell St. side and turn right. Where the Panhandle ends, turn left at Baker, then turn right at Hayes St. Alamo Square is three blocks up. Enter midway, about where Pierce St. hits Hayes, and climb up the gentle slope to the top of the park. It's a fairly conventional park, as San Francisco parks go—a hilly lawn with a grove of trees at its center, a single fenced-in tennis court—but the view from the park is a classic. Head over the crest and down the eastern slope and you'll spot the photographers. They're always here, snapping shots of the row of impeccable Victorian houses along Steiner St., with the downtown skyline beyond. It's a surefire cover shot—you'll have seen the image on scores of tourist brochures and guidebooks. The Victorian stars of this view, at 710–722 Steiner St., are notable mostly for their near uniformity and for being little changed over the years. They are not the most beautiful Victorians in the city or even on Alamo Square. The house at 1198 Fulton St., on the other side of the park, is much more striking but lacks the dramatic backdrop.

● Head down to Steiner St. and turn left. While crossing Fulton St. look to the right and you'll see the street descends directly toward City Hall. It's a perfect vantage point of the building's handsome, helmet-like dome. On the opposite corner, at 1000 Fulton, the huge house with the mansard roof is called the Archbishop's Mansion, because it was built in 1904 for Archbishop Riordan. It's a hotel now, and the Archbishop's old bedroom gets frequent use as a honeymoon suite.

● Continue on Steiner. At No. 1057, on the corner of Golden Gate Ave., the Chateau Tivoli is one of the city's most distinctive buildings. It jabs at the sky with a full complement of turrets and dainty weathervanes, which are the Victorian architectural equivalent of propeller caps. The building has some mighty alluring curves, especially around its bay windows. It was built in 1892 and has served in a variety of capacities, including as a rooming house during the 1960s and '70s. More recently it has been beautifully restored and converted into a hotel (with surprisingly reasonable rates). Walk on around the corner, where the adjacent apartment buildings (at 1409–1417 Golden Gate) are collectively known as the "Seattle Block." The buildings went up at the same time as the Tivoli, and are equally well preserved, and collectively they make a marvelous row.

● Turn left and follow Golden Gate to Divisadero St., where you can grab a refreshment at the BlueJay Cafe, a lunch and dinner spot that's good for comfort foods and beer. For a less-involved pit stop, head up to the corner of Folsom St. and snag a table at Cafe Abir, your basic coffeehouse with a laptoppin' crowd. Heading south on Divisadero will get you back to the Castro.

POINTS OF INTEREST

Archbishop's Mansion 1000 Fulton St., 415-563-7872

The Chateau Tivoli 1057 Steiner St., 415-776-5462

BlueJay Cafe 919 Divisadero St., 415-447-6066

Cafe Abir 1300 Fulton St., 415-567-7654

ROUTE SUMMARY

1. Start at the base of Corona Heights—at the top of Beaver St. or on the corner of 16th and Flint streets.
2. Follow the trail to the top of Corona Heights.
3. Head down through the dog run, exiting the park at the corner of Museum Way and Roosevelt St., and head up Roosevelt St.
4. Turn left at Park Hill.
5. At Buena Vista Ave. East, cross to the park and turn left on the sidewalk.
6. Head up the sand-and-wood steps, the first stairway to the right.
7. Find the asphalt path and follow it to the top.
8. Wandering through the park, find your way to the exit near the corner of Buena Vista Ave. West and Frederick St.
9. Turn right on Buena Vista Ave. West.
10. Cross Haight St. and continue on Central Ave.
11. Cross Oak St. to enter the Panhandle and turn right.
12. Turn left at Baker St.
13. Turn right at Hayes St.
14. Enter Alamo Square where Pierce St. meets Hayes St. and head up to the top.
15. Make your way down to Steiner St. and turn left.
16. Turn left at Golden Gate Ave. and follow it to Divisadero St.

View downtown from Corona Heights

Anza St

Parker Ave

Anzavista Ave
Turk Blvd

Turk Blvd

Golden Gate Ave

McAllister St

Scott St

Pierce St

Masonic Ave

Central Ave

Lyon St

Baker St

Broderick St

Alamo
Square

University of San Francisco

Willard St

McAllister St

Fulton St

Fulton St

Grove St

Hayes St

Scott St

Divisadero St

finish

Stanyan St

Shrader St

Cole St

Clayton St

Ashbury St

Fell St

Oak St

Fell St

The Panhandle

Page St

start

Golden
Gate
Park

Oak St

Page St

Haight St

Kezar Dr

Cole St

Haight St

Waller St

Buena
Vista
Park

Alpine Ter

Buena Vista Ter

Stanyan St

Beulah St

Cole St

Belvedere St

Waller St

Clayton St

Downey St

Ashbury St

Delmar St

Masonic Ave

Java St

Roosevelt Way

14th St

Castro St

Kezar Stadium

Frederick St

Upper Ter

15th St

Corona
Heights
Park

Flint St

Beaver St

Carl St

Clifford Ter

Levant St

Ord Ct

16th St

0   200   400   600 yards

0   200   400   600 meters

29 HaIGHT-aSHBURY: SaUNTERING BACK TO THE '60S

BOUNDARIES: **Scott St., Waller St., Fulton St., North Willard St.**
PARKING: **Unrestricted street parking can be found on Oak St., along the Panhandle.**
DISTANCE: **2 miles**
DIFFICULTY: **Easy**
PUBLIC TRANSIT: **N Judah streetcar (get off at Duboce Park); 24, 71 Muni buses**

Along with the Gold Rush, earthquakes, and the Gay '70s, the Summer of Love is one of those things for which San Francisco is commonly known to the outside world. The intersection of Haight and Ashbury streets is the city's most famous crossroads thanks to some craziness that occurred around this nexus from the mid- to late 1960s. While many hippies were simply indulging in the neighborhood's proliferation of drugs and sex, some idealistically saw the "Psychedelic Revolution" as hope for a better world. The neighborhood developed its own economy, spawned its own musical sound, and acquired a distinctive look, as its residents went for a shaggier, more colorful style than the rest of America. It must have been exciting, mind-blowing, and hilarious. If time travel were possible, Haight St. 1967 would be a tourist mecca. The street today does its best to live up to its reputation. Walking the neighborhood is a satisfying blend of historic sites, exquisite Victorian architecture, and bustling alternative commerce.

● We'll start on a nondescript corner, where Scott and Page streets meet. The building at 250 Scott, where Jack's Record Cellar is located, played a significant role in the neighborhood's countercultural past. The upstairs flat was the home of poet Kenneth Rexroth, a central player in the San Francisco Renaissance. This home-grown literary movement attracted the likes of Jack Kerouac and Allen Ginsberg to San Francisco, bringing the Beat movement to the city by the bay. The cafes of North Beach were the big draw, but the serious salons took place in Rexroth's pad. Rexroth distanced himself from the Beats, and moved East, but thousands of students and poets moved into the Haight, looking for cheap rents and an arty bohemian atmosphere in the decade before the hippies. The record shop is rarely open, but if it is, step in. It's San Francisco's oldest purveyor of collectible 33-, 45-, and 78-rpm records, and the shop's walls are covered with historic concert posters from legendary jazz, R&B, and rock shows.

● Head west on Page St. On the corner of Broderick St., at No. 1090, once stood the Albin Rooming House. According to rock historian Joel Selvin, this apartment building had a "ballroom" in the basement, where Big Brother and the Holding Company and other bands frequently performed. There's nothing to see here, except in your imagination, so keep a-moving.

● At the corner of Lyon St. turn right. The attractive Victorian at No. 112 was the home of singer Janis Joplin during the Summer of Love. It was an apartment house in those days, and Joplin's room was on the second floor with the curved balcony off the front.

● Head north one block to Oak St. and cross into the Panhandle, a shady, pencil-thin green that's ideal for dog-walking. Exciting events took place here during the '60s, including unforgettable free outdoor concerts. Jimi Hendrix once played here, so as you walk a block west in the park imagine his awesome sound reverberating off the apartment buildings along either side.

● At Central Ave. turn left and at Haight St. turn right. On this block you'll see two relics of the Haight's radical past. The Bound Together Book Collective, at No. 1369, has been peddling anarchist treatises since 1976. Pipe Dreams, at No. 1376, is the oldest extant head shop on the strip. Stop by for an armful of bongs, hookahs, tobacco products, and groovy patches for your torn Levi's.

● At the end of the block, the Magnolia Pub & Brewery is an attractive corner noshery that features its own home-brewed ales. The façade is little changed since the '60s, when the site was the Drogstore Cafe. The name was an obvious appeal to the drug culture, with a twist in the spelling to throw the cops off the scent. Today, some lovely cask ales are produced in the pub's basement and pumped up directly through the taps on the bar. Good pub food, too.

● Across Masonic Ave., Positively Haight Street is a garish grotto of grooviness. The shop deals in everything you'll need for that '60s flashback you've been meaning to have—from tie-dye shirts and incense to loose-fitting imports from India. If none of that's your bag, you can always admire the building's far-out exterior, with its columns shaped like Desi Arnaz congas and cartoony mural work on the window trim.

- A block up, the corner of Ashbury is the epicenter of the neighborhood. Snap some shots of the crisscrossing Haight and Ashbury street signs and hang a louie. Past Waller St., the Victorian at 710 Ashbury was the home of the Grateful Dead as the band reached its prime (back in the days when bands conveniently lived together, like characters in a TV sitcom). Jerry Garcia, Bob Weir, and Pigpen lived in the psychedelic frat house with managers Rock Scully and Danny Rifkin from 1966 to 1968. Snap a few shots of the house, now home to unfamous millionaires, and beat it on back to Haight.

- Make a left on Ashbury, where half a block up, at 1568 Haight, is Martin Mack's, a standard-issue fake Irish pub. In the late '60s, it was the Pall Mall Lounge, where the "Love Burgers" were very popular, most likely because if you didn't have any scratch you could have yours free of charge. Across the street, at No. 1599, Soul Patch Tattoo and Piercing keeps some of the neighborhood spirit alive. If permanent body art is too much of a commitment, you can get a henna tattoo that'll last just a while.

- Past Clayton St., the Red Victorian is another standard-bearer for the old neighborhood. It's a gorgeous old inn, built in 1904. Inside, it's positively kooky. Owner Sami Sunchild, now well over 80, designed all the guest rooms to induce drug-free hallucinations. She hangs more of her trippy art in a gallery off the lobby, so feel free to have a look inside. The people are friendly, as is right for a place calling itself a "world peace center." They hold a variety of peace-related programming, including the "Sunday Morning Breakfast Conversations," which are open to locals and travelers. Across the street, take a look at Wasteland, a vintage clothing emporium. The Beaux Arts façade is an eyeful.

- The Goodwill store on the corner of Haight and Cole streets was the site of the Straight Theater in 1967 and '68. Legendary shows took place here, and the Dead often used the hall as a rehearsal space. Across the street, at 1775 Haight, the Diggers kept a "crash pad," where anyone needing a free place to sleep could come. The Diggers provided free food and clothing as well. It later turned out that actor Peter Coyote was among the organization's anonymous leaders.

victorian Detours

While Haight St. is the wigged-out main stem of the neighborhood, you'd be missing the flip side of the area's charm if you didn't take a few short detours to admire some of San Francisco's finest residential architecture. You'll find gems concentrated on the 1700 block of Oak (between Ashbury and Clayton), the 400 block of Clayton (between Oak and Page), the 500 block of Cole (between Page and Haight), and the 1900 block of Page (between Shrader and Stanyan).

- Near Shrader St., Kan Zaman is a way-out eatery serving Palestinian and Lebanese food while belly dancers gyrate on the dining room floor. You can also puff on a hookah here. The shisha blends are legal and likely to make you only a little dizzy.

- Next block, in a converted bowling alley, is the immense Amoeba Music, one of the city's best shopping stops for music. On many an early evening free, live shows are held in the store.

- Turn right at Stanyan St., walk along the eastern edge of Golden Gate Park, and turn left at Fulton St. We're looking for the Jefferson Airplane mansion, at No. 2400. It's a block up, at the corner of North Willard, the end of your walk. It's a truly impressive three-story manse with a neoclassic columned entry. Members of the band moved here in 1968, painted the place black, and stayed through the 1970s. Along the way, the Airplane was converted into a Starship. Singer Grace Slick left San Francisco for a bigger galaxy (Los Angeles) in the early '80s, saying she was tired of being a big fish in a small pond.

POINTS OF INTEREST

Bound Together Book Collective 1369 Haight St., 415-431-8355

Pipe Dreams 1376 Haight St., 415-431-3553

Magnolia Pub & Brewery 1398 Haight St., 415-864-7468

Positively Haight Street 1400 Haight St., 415-252-8747

Soul Patch Tattoo and Piercing 1599 Haight St., 415-552-3444

Wasteland 1660 Haight St., 415-863-3150

Red Victorian B&B 1665 Haight St., 415-864-1978

Kan Zaman 1793 Haight St., 415-751-9656

Amoeba Music 1855 Haight St., 415-831-1200

ROUTE SUMMARY

1. Start at the corner of Scott and Page streets.
2. Walk west on Page St.
3. Turn right at Lyon St.
4. At Oak St., cross into the Panhandle and walk west for one block.
5. Turn left at Central Ave.
6. Turn right at Haight St.
7. Turn left at Ashbury St. and walk a block and a half to No. 710, then return to Haight St.
8. Turn left at Haight St.
9. Turn right at Stanyan St.
10. Turn left at Fulton St.
11. Stop at the corner of Fulton and Willard streets.

Positively Haight Street

PACIFIC
OCEAN

WALK 30 GOLDEN GATE PARK

China Beach

The Presidio

Mountain Lake Park

Clay St

Lincoln Park

Lake St

California St

Clement St

Geary Blvd

Euclid Ave

Clement St

Geary Blvd

Balboa St

Cabrillo St

Cabrillo St

Fulton St

Fulton St

Anza St

Arguello Blvd

Stanyan St

Parker Ave

finish

Spreckels Lake

Polo Field

Lloyd Lake

Golden Gate Park

Stow Lake

Lily Pond

start

Kezar Stadium

Lincoln Way

South Dr

Lincoln Way

Irving St

Irving St

Judah St

Carl St

Kirkham St

Moraga St

Noriega St

Ortega St

Pacheco St

Quintara St

Quintara St

Great Hwy

Sunset Blvd

0   500   1000   1500 yards

0   500   1000   1500 meters

32nd Ave · 30th Ave · 27th Ave · 25th Ave · 26th Ave · 24th Ave · 21st Ave · 18th Ave · 16th Ave · 15th Ave · Park Presidio · 12th Ave · 11th Ave · 10th Ave · 8th Ave · 6th Ave · 3rd Ave · 4th Ave

47th Ave · 45th Ave · 43rd Ave · 41st Ave · 38th Ave · 36th Ave · 34th Ave

48th Ave · 46th Ave · 44th Ave · 42nd Ave · 40th Ave · 38th Ave · 33rd Ave · 31st Ave · 29th Ave · 28th Ave · 26th Ave · 24th Ave · 23rd Ave · 22nd Ave · 21st Ave · 20th Ave · 19th Ave · 18th Ave · 17th Ave · 10th Ave · 9th Ave · 7th Ave · 5th Ave · 3rd Ave

41st Ave

30 GOLDEN GATE PARK: A LOT OF PARK (AND SOME DANDY MUSEUMS)

BOUNDARIES: **Stanyan St., Fulton St., Lincoln Way, Great Highway**
DISTANCE: **4½ miles**
DIFFICULTY: **Moderate (no great hills, but it's a long, indirect route through a huge park)**
PARKING: **Street parking is easier to find on weekdays than on weekends. The underground lot by the De Young Museum is reached via the 8th Ave. entrance, on the north side of the park.**
PUBLIC TRANSIT: **N Judah streetcar; 6, 33, 71 Muni buses**

Golden Gate Park is a celebration of nature—only, there is really nothing natural about it. The 1,000-acre urban parkland, among the nation's largest, is a series of groves, gardens, and lakes, all seeded, shaped, and constructed by human hands and machinery. When the city set aside the land, in 1870, it was a windswept expanse of sand and shrubs that few thought could be tamed for the leisurely enjoyment of the local citizenry. William Hammond Hall, the park's surveyor and first superintendent, planted barley, and then lupine, both of which rooted and spread across the sands, holding it down and making it possible for further planting to take place. Within ten years, natural-looking woodlands had been established across the once-barren land. The park also has historic buildings, museums, a boathouse, a bison paddock, and a classy brewpub. Plan on spending a few hours walking and exploring the terrain before enjoying a well-earned beer or meal.

● **Start at McLaren Lodge, near the convergence of Stanyan St. and John F. Kennedy Dr. This lodge-like graystone, with Moorish-Gothic overtones, was built in 1896 and serves as the park's headquarters (but it offers only limited information to visitors). It is named for John McLaren, the park superintendent from 1890 until 1947—an astonishing run of 57 years that ended with McLaren's death at age 97. Clearly, the guy was as sturdy as an ox.**

● **Follow JFK Dr. into the park, and on the right-hand side you'll soon see the Conservatory of Flowers, a grand glass house constructed in 1876. It's the oldest** structure in the park. Making a brief visit is well worth the $7 admission charge. The humid interior is a welcome contrast with the park's typical blustery weather, making the conservatory a suitable home for the varied and exotic tropical plants housed within.

● From the conservatory, cross JFK and look for the 20-foot-tall ferns. Follow the dirt path through this Jurassic-looking grove, veering left at the fork. You'll quickly reach secluded Lily Pond, which the trail loops partway around as it leads to Middle Dr. East. See if you can spot the unofficial trails leading to hidden homeless camps within some of the dense growth here and in other parts of the park.

● Cross Middle Dr. East and turn left (east), looking for the entrance to the National AIDS Memorial Grove. Designated by an Act of Congress, the grove is a reflective place where people can think of loved ones lost to AIDS. Memorial services are often held here, and a stone patio along the path, called Circle of Friends, has names of some victims etched in an ever-widening spiral. From here, the path leads by a stand of young redwoods and through a grassy dell and alongside an artfully landscaped dry creek. Past that, by a meditative circle, look for stone steps to the left and head up. When you reach the asphalt path, head left, then right where a dirt path heads downhill. (This should all be fairly easy to follow when you're actually on the trail.) Sticking to the main path downhill will get you through a stone garden, and then a baseball field will come into view. Veer back toward Middle Dr. East and turn left.

● Veer right at Martin Luther King Jr. Dr. When you see the sign for Shakespeare Garden, follow it and you'll soon reach the Music Concourse; turn right. Here you'll see the new California Academy of Sciences, the De Young Museum, the huge band shell called the Temple of Music, and the Japanese Tea Garden. Walk through the concourse.

The concourse area was laid out for the 1894 Midwinter International Exposition, commonly described as a chintzy flop, but looking pretty interesting if photographs from the time are any indication. Some 200 temporary structures filled the grounds, many of them reflecting the pretentious and exotic tastes of San Franciscans at the time. The city was eager to make a big impression on more established bigwigs of the East Coast and Chicago.

In any case, all that survives from the expo is the Japanese Village, now called the Japanese Tea Garden. After the expo, stewardship of the gardens was turned over to Makoto Hagiwara, who built a house on the grounds and lived here with his family. Hagiwara was fired in 1900, rehired in 1907, and stayed on until he was interned along with thousands of Japanese immigrants during World War II. Hagiwara's other contribution to the local culture was the introduction of fortune cookies (apparently invented by his cook in 1914), which were originally made as a unique snack to serve at the Tea Garden but are now ubiquitous in Chinese restaurants.

The California Academy of Sciences reopened in 2008, its four-story rain forest and its living roof sparking much fanfare and attracting lines down the sidewalk and beyond the concourse. Things have calmed considerably, but a visit still requires a few hours, so save it for another time.

- The De Young Museum opened in 2005, initially to mixed reviews that have warmed since. San Franciscans are always a little suspicious of modern architecture, especially bold designs like this one, with its askew, 144-foot tower prominent above the park's treetops. It's clad in unprotected copper, which has begun acquiring a patina that's very easy on the eyes. Admission is $10, which deters quick in-and-out visits. The De Young's art collection and exhibits warrant a follow-up visit, so let's keep walking.

- Turn left on Hagiwara Tea Garden Dr. and walk back out to MLK, cross the street, and enter the Strybing Arboretum via the Friend Gate. The arboretum is another site worth a dedicated visit, with 70 acres showcasing some 7,500 varieties of plants from around the world. Its labyrinth of paths are tempting to get lost in. For the purpose of our westward trek, take every right turn and you'll end up at an exit a little ways farther down MLK.

- Just outside the arboretum, look across the street for stone steps, which lead to Stow Lake, and head up. At the top of the steps, turn left on the shaded path, which clings to the water's edge. The lake here is a narrow ring, looking like a calm stream looped around high Strawberry Hill. You'll see plenty of paddle boats and ducks. When you reach the rustic stone bridge, cross and turn right, following the inside of the curvature of the lake. Soon after you pass the Chinese Pavilion, looking like a gazebo awaiting a tea party, you'll hear and then see Huntington Falls, a charming artifice. This is perhaps the only part of the park where the hush of city traffic is completely drowned out, making it worth pausing for a little break here. Continue along the trail to Roman Bridge, cross it, and head left toward the boathouse. Behind the boathouse a trail leads to JFK Dr. Turn left.

● After crossing Cross Over Dr. and Transverse Dr., look for the footpath to the left of JFK. You'll be walking past a wooded area to the left and picnic grounds and large green meadows to the right. Speedway Meadow has been the site of many an outdoor concert, including the immensely popular Hardly Strictly Bluegrass Festival, which takes place every October. The trail leads to the Polo Field, which is surrounded by a "trotting track" for equestrians. Golden Gate Park Stables are across the Polo Field. The field is not so much known for polo matches as it is for the cultural events that have taken place here. On the afternoon of January 14, 1967, the Summer of Love got off to an early start here, with the Gathering of the Tribes and Human Be-In. Some 30,000 hippies congregated here to follow Timothy Leary's call to "Turn on, tune in, drop out." Allen Ginsberg ranted, the Grateful Dead jammed, and the crowd tripped late into the night. When the Dead's Jerry Garcia died in August 1995, a spontaneous gathering took place in the Polo Field as fans instinctively came here to remember the keeper of the '60s flame.

● Beyond the stables, a path leads back to JFK Dr., where you turn left. On the other side, you'll see the Bison Paddock. Golden Gate Park has no zoo and is more about flora than fauna, but a herd of buffalo has lived here since 1892.

● Follow JFK around the golf course. Before the street ends at the Great Highway, the Dutch Windmill overlooks a garden of tulips. The windmill was built in 1902 to pump water into the park. It was restored in the early 1980s and still works. There's another windmill at the southwest corner of the park, but it's in a sad state of disrepair.

● The Beach Chalet stands a the corner of JFK and the Great Highway. Designed by Willis Polk, the restaurant opened in 1925. The downstairs lobby is covered with murals, painted in 1936 by French-born artist Lucien Labaudt. Upstairs, in a room dominated by plate-glass windows facing the ocean, the microbrewery is a lively spot for breakfast, lunch, or dinner. The beer is good, and on many evenings live jazz combos perform. Alternatively, immediately behind the Beach Chalet, Park Chalet features small-plate California cuisine, indoor-outdoor seating, and often shorter waits for a table.

POINTS OF INTEREST

Conservatory of Flowers John F. Kennedy Dr., 415-666-7001

Hagiwara Japanese Tea Garden Hagiwara Tea Garden Dr., 415-831-2700

California Academy of Sciences 55 Music Concourse Dr., 415-379-8000

M.H. De Young Memorial Museum 50 Hagiwara Tea Garden Dr., 415-863-3330

Strybing Arboretum & Botanical Gardens 9th Ave. at Lincoln Way, 415-661-1316

Beach Chalet and Park Chalet 1000 Great Highway, 415-386-8439

Conservatory of Flowers

route summary

1. Begin at the John McLaren Lodge, at the intersection of Stanyan St. and John F. Kennedy Dr.
2. Follow JFK Dr. to the Conservatory of Flowers.
3. Opposite the conservatory, follow the dirt trail through the fern grove.
4. Follow the trail halfway around Lily Pond.
5. Where the trail hits Middle Dr. East, turn left.
6. At Middle Dr. and Bowling Green Dr., enter the AIDS Memorial Grove.
7. Follow the path through the AIDS Memorial Grove.
8. A series of dirt and asphalt paths will lead to the ball field. If you get lost, just follow Middle Dr. East in a westerly direction.
9. At Martin Luther King Jr. Dr., turn right.
10. Past the Shakespeare Garden, turn right at the entry to the Music Concourse and walk through it, to Hagiwara Tea Garden Dr.
11. Turn left at Tea Garden Dr. to return to MLK Dr.
12. Across MLK Dr., enter the Strybing Arboretum and turn right.
13. In the arboretum, veer right where trails meet and you'll end up farther up MLK.
14. Cross MLK Dr. and head up the stone steps to Stow Lake.
15. Turn left onto the trail.
16. Cross Rustic Bridge and turn right.
17. Cross Roman Bridge and turn left.
18. Behind the boathouse follow the trail to JFK Dr. and turn left.
19. Past Transverse Dr. get on the footpath and follow it past Speedway Meadow, all the way to the Polo Field.
20. Loop partway around the Polo Field (or diagonally across it) to the stables.
21. Behind the stables, find your way back to JFK Dr. and turn left.
22. Follow JFK Dr. as it bends in a northwest direction all the way to the Beach Chalet.

Fern Grove

Sacramento St

California St

Buchanan St

Pine St

Webster St

Gough St

Orben Pl

Pine St

Austin St

Octavia St

Bush St

Fillmore St

Wilmot St

Laguna St

Bush St

Sutter St

Cottage Row

Sutter St

Hemlock St

Post St

Webster St

Peace Plaza

Geary Blvd

finish

Japan Center

Zampa Ln

Steiner St

Geary Blvd

start

Western Shore Ln

Cleary Ct

Fillmore St

O'Farrell St

Hollis St

Inca Ln

Byington St

| 0 | 100 | 200 | 300 yards |
| 0 | 100 | 200 | 300 meters |

31 JaPantown and Fillmore Street: where BUDDHIST TeMPLeS AND BLUeS BarS Meet

BOUNDARIES: **Fillmore St., Geary Blvd., Pine St., Octavia St.**
DISTANCE: **1¼ miles**
DIFFICULTY: **Easy**
PARKING: **There is a parking lot beneath Japan Center. Street parking is often available on Webster St., south of Geary Blvd.**
PUBLIC TRANSIT: **The 22 and 38 Muni buses stop at the corner of Geary Blvd. and Fillmore St.**

Japantown is an odd and interesting neighborhood. Japanese immigrants began settling here after the '06 quake and were unjustly moved from their homes and relocated in internment camps during World War II. The African Americans who moved in were drawn by jobs in wartime industries, but 1960s redevelopment of the area caused yet another exodus as a sizeable proportion of the neighborhood's housing was demolished to make way for the widened Geary Blvd. Expressway and for hotels and retail structures. Although the Japanese had dispersed by that time, the redevelopment included construction of Japan Center, along with some senior housing catering to elderly Japanese. So what we have here is a modern commercial district with a strong Japanese flavor and only a very small remnant of the Japanese community. Similarly, Fillmore St. retains hints of the area's African-American past. Amid the modern hotels and condominiums are some gorgeous Victorians that were spared the mid-century wrecking ball. The neighborhood is pleasant for walking, but the chief interest here is inside Japan Center itself. We'll end up there.

● **Start at the southwest corner of Geary Blvd. and Fillmore St., at the Fillmore Auditorium, legendary for its rock shows during the 1960s. The elegant hall predates rock and roll by several decades, however. It was built in 1912 and was originally dubbed the Majestic Ball Room. Very likely some of the most remarkable shows to ever take place in the building were by jazz and R&B performers during the heyday of the black Fillmore District. Count Basie, Billie Holliday, and a young James Brown electrified audiences here. Rock promoter Bill Graham put on shows here from 1966** to 1968. All the local bands (Dead, Airplane, Holding Company) took the stage on a regular basis, and out-of-town guests included Jimi Hendrix, the Doors, and the Velvet Underground. The Fillmore re-established itself as one of the city's preeminent rock venues in the 1990s and remains an intimate venue where top-tier talent performs in a variety of musical styles.

● Cross Geary Blvd. to reach the Boom Boom Room, a Fillmore District stalwart. This classy little cinderblock dive was for many years known as Jack's. It's a lounge-like, inner-city juke, with black-and-white checkered linoleum floor, padded booths, and a small stage where blues artists perform nightly. During the late 1990s, the club was partly owned by bluesman John Lee Hooker, who for many years lived in Redwood City, just south of San Francisco. Hooker died in 2001.

● Cross Fillmore St. at Post St. On the ground floor of the purple Victorian at No. 1712, Marcus Books specializes in literature by black writers. The house itself was moved here during the 1960s, as were many other homes during the redevelopment of the neighborhood. In its earlier location, on Post St. where the Buchanan St. Mall is now, this house was home to Jimbo's Bop City, a music locus in the old Fillmore where the likes of Charlie Parker joined in after-hours jams.

● Turn right on Sutter St. and walk on the north (right-hand) side of the street. Before reaching Webster St., head up the path called Cottage Row. The six two-story cottages along this little pedestrian block were built in 1882. Cottage Row ends at Bush St. Turn right and right again on Webster. At No. 1737, the John J. Vollmer House is one of the neighborhood's better-surviving Victorians. Built in 1885, it was moved here in the mid-1970s. It was evidently a tight fit—part of the house had to be sliced off to get it into the narrow lot. Nevertheless, the trim, with flowers carved into the woodwork, is some of the city's finest.

● Turn left on Sutter and left on Laguna St. At 1909 Bush St. is the Konko Church, where members of a sect of the Shinto religion worship. The church, built in a simple yet graceful Japanese style, went up in 1973.

● Turn right on Pine St. Just off the corner of Octavia St., at 1881 Pine, the large structure with the stupa on the roof is the home of the Buddhist Church. The temple was built in 1937, but the Jodo Shinshu congregation began worshipping here, in an earlier building, in 1914. Hidden within the stupa are relics of the Buddha, given to the congregation by the Emperor of Thailand in 1935.

● Turn right on Octavia. At Bush, the corner lot behind the row of eucalyptus trees on the Octavia St. side is of historical interest. In the 1860s Mary Ellen Pleasant built her house here. Pleasant caused quite a stir in San Francisco more or less by being a black woman who enjoyed tremendous success here. From surviving photos, she appears to have been a very serious and intelligent woman who probably took no guff from anyone. But the house she built here became known as the "House of Mystery," after her business partner and assumed lover Thomas Bell died here under suspicious circumstances. Local papers never seemed to know how to deal with this woman, and generally implied she was a voodoo priestess of some kind. In fact, she was from Philadelphia and for decades aided slaves escaping via the Underground Railroad. Even in San Francisco she often harbored black fugitives, all the while amassing her fortune by operating a string of well-regarded boarding houses and investing in the stock market and real estate. She died in 1904 and her mansion was destroyed in 1927. There's a plaque embedded in the sidewalk, amid the eucalyptus trees.

● Continue on Octavia and turn right on Sutter St. At Buchanan turn left into the Buchanan St. Mall, a pedestrian shopping strip that echoes the Asian emphasis of Japan Center, to which the street directly leads. Japan Center was built in the 1960s, and architecturally it reflects the style of the era but with distinct Japanese overtones. It was designed by Minoru Yamasaki, who went on to achieve greater heights by designing the ill-fated World Trade Center in New York. A 100-foot pagoda stands in Peace Plaza, a stark concrete slab where the elderly sometimes take in some sun. To the left is the Hotel Kabuki, a very fashionable hostelry in which the rooms have sleek Japanese stylings. To the right is Kintetsu Mall. Go on in.

● The mall has the meandering feel of an airport, with food courts and narrow stores selling the same sorts of cultural curios you'd find in duty-free shops. If the impulse strikes you, you might wind up with a new silk kimono while here. Of more likely interest is the Kinokuniya Bookstore, where several aisles are devoted to Japanese art books, Manga comics, DVDs of anime films, and a smattering of Godzilla classics.

On your way there, you'll pass through the restaurant mall, where the decor really lays it on with the movie-set Japantown feel. The windows all have artfully arranged plastic meals on display to lure you in. Mifune is a good spot for a bowl of hot udon soup. The mall also has several cafes, the posh Sundance Kabuki Cinemas (with a bar, a bistro, and a restaurant within it), and karaoke bars, if you're planning on hanging out awhile. Downstairs, accessible via Post St. near the corner of Webster, be sure to drop by the Nijiya Market, a supermarket in miniature, with tiny carts and narrow aisles stocked with Japanese foodstuffs. Just past the registers, an aisle is stocked with a huge selection of bento lunches neatly packed in plastic trays.

POINTS OF INTEREST

Fillmore Auditorium 1805 Geary Blvd., 415-346-6000

Boom Boom Room 1601 Fillmore St., 415-673-8000

Marcus Books 1712 Fillmore St., 415-346-4222

Konko Kyo Church 1909 Bush St.

Buddhist Church 1881 Pine St.

Hotel Kabuki 1625 Post St., 415-922-3200

Kinokuniya Bookstore 1581 Webster St., 415-567-7625

Sundance Kabuki Cinemas, 1881 Post St., 415-346-3243

Nijiya Market 1737 Post St., 415-563-1901

route summary

1. Start at the Fillmore Auditorium on the southwest corner of Geary Blvd. and Fillmore St.
2. Proceed north on Fillmore St.
3. Turn right on Sutter St. and walk half a block on the north side of the street.
4. Turn left on Cottage Row (pedestrian street).
5. Turn right on Bush St.
6. Turn right on Webster St.
7. Turn left on Sutter St.
8. Turn left on Laguna St.
9. Turn right on Pine St.
10. Turn right on Octavia St.
11. Turn right on Sutter St.
12. Turn left on Buchanan St. (pedestrian mall).
13. Cross Post St. to Peace Plaza.
14. To the right, enter Kintetsu Mall.

Peace Pagoda

The Presidio

Pacific Ave

Mountain Lake

Mountain Lake Park

Lincoln Blvd

Hays

Lake St

5th Ave

4th Ave

3rd Ave

Arguello Blvd

Cornwall St

21st Ave

20th Ave

19th Ave

Lake St

14th Ave

Funston Ave

12th Ave

11th Ave

10th Ave

California St

Clement St

start

Clement St

23rd Ave

24th Ave

Clement St

18th Ave

17th Ave

16th Ave

15th Ave

5th Ave

4th Ave

3rd Ave

2nd Ave

Arguello Blvd

finish

Geary Blvd

Anza St

Funston Ave

Park Presidio

8th Ave

7th Ave

6th Ave

Anza St

Balboa St

25th Ave

24th Ave

23rd Ave

22nd Ave

Balboa St

18th Ave

17th Ave

16th Ave

14th Ave

12th Ave

11th Ave

10th Ave

9th Ave

Cabrillo St

Cabrillo St

Cabrillo St

1

Fulton St

Golden Gate Park

0   200   400   600 yards
0   200   400   600 meters

32 richmond district: an international stroll

BOUNDARIES: **Arguello St., Clement St., Geary Blvd., 25th Ave.**
DISTANCE: **1½ miles**
DIFFICULTY: **Easy**
PARKING: **Street parking is metered, with two-hour limits. Parking is very difficult to find on the weekend.**
PUBLIC TRANSIT: **1, 38 Muni buses**

Clement St. in the Inner Richmond District will always be "New Chinatown," even though Chinese immigrants have operated businesses here since the 1970s. The area naturally invites contrast to the old Chinatown, and indeed there are interesting similarities and differences. Being out in San Francisco's Fog Belt, Richmond has always attracted more than its share of immigrants, and there's plenty of evidence of many waves of newcomers, some of whom are obviously still here. To be sure, along Clement you'll find roasted ducks hanging in windows, along with steamed pork buns, produce stalls, and bargain bazaars to rival, if not surpass, those of the old Chinatown. But in the mix you'll also encounter the city's best used bookstore, Russian tearooms, Korean barbecue joints, Irish bars, bohemian cafes, and loads of Southeast Asian restaurants. This walk is sort of an eating and shopping excursion that needn't involve maxing out your credit card. The main idea is to snoop around a bit to see what sorts of intriguing items you might find along one of the city's more interesting streets.

● Begin at the end of Clement St., on the corner of Arguello Blvd., and go west. If the fog is blowing the other way, you'll know you're headed in the right direction. If it's daytime the Plough and the Stars, at No. 116, will not be open, which is just as well as we aim to get a little walking done. Note that this is no fake Irish pub, which should be apparent from the bar's exterior, which doesn't bother to project a St. Paddy's Day party atmosphere. Instead, the place has genuine spirit. Irish musicians perform here every night, and many of the patrons come to do a little fancy steppin'.

● A block up, at No. 208, is Minh's Garden, where perfectly passable Vietnamese food is served. Better yet, on the next block, at No. 309, is Burma Super Star. Despite the Hollywood leanings of its name, Burma Super Star is a fairly humble place that serves a type of cuisine not commonly found in the U.S. The food of Myanmar is

Back Story: The San Francisco Columbarium

While exploring Clement St. in the Inner Richmond District, it's worth a quick detour to check out the San Francisco Columbarium. It's one of those places San Franciscans hear about but never get around to visiting, and it's just a couple of blocks from where this tour begins.

A columbarium is a building divided into compartments in which the ashes of the dead can be kept. The word derives from the Latin *columba,* meaning "dove," and is a reference to the tightly arranged coops built for domesticated doves and pigeons. That's not particularly flattering. In general, it might be appropriate to think of columbaria as old folks' homes for folks who are just a wee bit beyond old. The San Francisco Columbarium, built in 1898, is a particularly elegant example. It's a gorgeous piece of historic architecture with beautiful tiling and graceful glass enclosures rising three stories above the main floor.

San Francisco is a city nearly devoid of cemeteries. Only two graveyards remain in the city—in the Presidio and behind Mission Dolores. Large cemeteries formerly covered much of the Inner Richmond, and the Columbarium was within the 167-acre Odd Fellows Cemetery. During the early 20th century all of these graveyards were moved south of San Francisco to the strange city of Colma, where the dead vastly outnumber the living. Thus, for the most part, San Francisco keeps the dearly departed at arm's length. The Columbarium was spared, even though cremation was for several decades outlawed in the city. It was restored in the late 1970s.

The Columbarium is the only place within the city limits where a civilian can hope to rest in peace. Vaults are privately owned, and their value rises and falls (mostly rises) with more energy than San Francisco's housing market. Annually, the Columbarium throws a cocktail party for people who own but do not yet occupy vaults. It's a way for future neighbors to get to know each other before they meet their makers.

The Columbarium is just a few blocks from Clement and Arguello streets. On Aguello walk two blocks south, past Geary Blvd., and turn left onto Anza St. Turn left onto Lorain Court, a cul-de-sac that ends at the entrance to the Columbarium.

spicy and aromatic, with rich curries and sizzling vegetables bringing together the influences of both East and South Asia. Sure enough, this little joint is very popular.

- On the next corner, Toy Boat Dessert Cafe is an ice cream parlor. While you're waiting for your server to scrape those scoops for you, check out the store's amusing array of toys and novelty items. They still sell Pez dispensers and Peewee Herman dolls here.

- Enough food. Kamei Housewares and Restaurant Supplies takes up two buildings, each filled to the rafters with utilitarian crockery, knives, bamboo placemats, chopsticks "for special guests," soup bowls, rice bowls, clay pots, and teapots.

- Across the street, Green Apple Books and Music is a large emporium of new and used books. It's a densely packed series of rooms both upstairs and down, with additional space a little ways down the block. Some patrons have been known to simply disappear here, never to be seen again.

- New May Wah Supermarket, at No. 719, is the sort of place you expect to find in a Chinatown-type of environment. It has an endless aisle devoted to Asian snacks—shrimp puffs, Pocky Sticks, and the like—and other rows fully stocked with bean sauces, fish sauces, and canned tropical fruits of the kind that aren't grown in the States (rambutan, longans, lychees, etc.). Take a gander.

- Wander out past Park Presidio Blvd. and you're committing yourself to a fairly long walk (unless you hop on a No. 38 bus for the return trip). Make a left on Park Presidio, cut over to Geary Blvd., and follow it all the way out to 25th Ave., and you might find yourself wanting to move out this way. Places you ought to look out for are Kabuto Sushi, at 5121 Geary, a fine and nondescript sushi restaurant. A few blocks farther, Ton Kiang, at No. 5821, prepares outstanding dim sum in an unfrenzied atmosphere (you select your dim sum from a menu, and it is prepared to order). Tommy's Mexican Restaurant, at No. 5929, is as well known for its margaritas as it is for its fine Yucatecan cuisine. The drinks are prepared by hand (no mixes) with high-quality tequila and fresh ingredients. The food goes down mighty easy after one or two of 'em.

- Tiki bars are all the rage around the Bay Area these days. They're throwbacks to the 1930s, when mainlanders first discovered ukulele music and longed for the easy life under South Seas palm trees. Trad'r Sam, at No. 6150, is no throwback. It's been operating out here in the fog since before World War II. It has all the atmosphere of Mr. and Mrs. Howell's hut, and fruity drinks prepared by hard-working barkeeps resemble Carmen Miranda's hats. Show up in the afternoon if you want to avoid the just-turned-21 crowd.

POINTS OF INTEREST

The Plough and the Stars 116 Clement St., 415-751-1122

Minh's Garden 208 Clement St., 415-751-8211

Burma Super Star 309 Clement St., 415-387-2147

Toy Boat Dessert Cafe 401 Clement St., 415-751-7505

Kamei Housewares and Restaurant Supplies 525–547 Clement St., 415-666-3688

Green Apple Books and Music 506 Clement St., 415-387-2272

New May Wah Supermarket 719 Clement St., 415-221-9826

Kabuto Sushi 5121 Geary Blvd., 415-752-5652

Ton Kiang 5821 Geary Blvd., 415-386-8530

Tommy's Mexican Restaurant 5929 Geary Blvd., 415-387-4747

Trad'r Sam 6150 Geary Blvd., 415-221-0773

San Francisco Columbarium 1 Loraine Court

ROUTE SUMMARY

1. Start at the Arguello Blvd. end of Clement St. and proceed west.
2. Turn left at Park Presidio Blvd.
3. Turn right at Geary Blvd.

Kamei on Clement Street

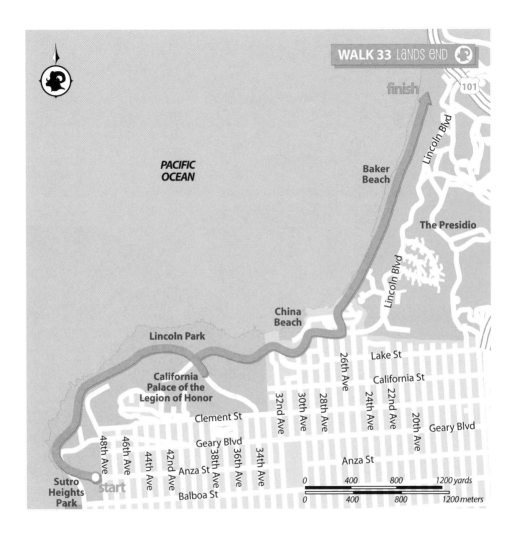

finish

101

PACIFIC
OCEAN

Lincoln Blvd

Baker
Beach

The Presidio

Lincoln Blvd

China
Beach

Lincoln Blvd

Lincoln Park

Lake St

26th Ave

California St

California
Palace of the
Legion of Honor

32nd Ave

30th Ave

28th Ave

24th Ave

22nd Ave

20th Ave

Clement St

Geary Blvd

34th Ave

Geary Blvd

48th Ave

46th Ave

44th Ave

42nd Ave

38th Ave

36th Ave

Anza St

Anza St

Sutro
Heights
Park

start

Balboa St

0   400   800   1200 yards

0   400   800   1200 meters

33 LaNDS END: CLIFFSIDE ParKS ON THE EDGE

BOUNDARIES: **48th Ave., Geary St., and the edge of the continent**
DISTANCE: **3 miles**
DIFFICULTY: **Strenuous (a bit hazardous in spots)**
PARKING: **Street parking on 48th Ave. near the end of Geary or Anza has no time limit.**
PUBLIC TRANSIT: **38 Muni bus**

San Francisco is oriented toward its bay, but to overlook the coastal trails that run along the cliffs at the city's western edge is to miss out on some very striking natural scenery. Trails, some of them slim and rocky footpaths, crook down to secluded beaches and back up to landmark buildings such as the Cliff House and the Palace of the Legion of Honor. The area's intriguing history manifests itself in captivating ways. The washed-out remnants of Sutro Baths are a modern ruin looking much like the leavings of a long-gone civilization. Be aware that nudity is tolerated on some of the beaches, so the natural scenery you encounter along the more secluded trails may include humans in their birthday suits. Take this walk on a cold day if you want to avoid such surprises.

● Begin at Sutro Heights Park, where once stood the estate of Adolf Sutro (see box). Sutro was an unusually civic-minded millionaire who fashioned his gardens into a grand park open to the public. He had the grounds landscaped in the style of an Italian garden, and although some cracked wise about Sutro's unrefined taste in art, San Franciscans seldom objected to the plaster nymph statues that peered out between the trees and shrubbery. All is gone now, save for some cypress trees, lovely rolling lawns, and what appears to be the broken footprint of Sutro's old manor house, which fell into disrepair after his death and was demolished in 1939. Beside a little gazebo-like structure, take the path that leads down to Point Lobos Ave. and the seaside cliffs.

● Cross the street and make your way down to the Cliff House. There have been several Cliff Houses on this site, beginning in 1863. The first Cliff House was owned by a retired sea captain known as Pop Foster, and for a time, Foster's Cliff House was known as a house of ill repute. Adolf Sutro bought the remote resort in the 1890s, it burned down in 1894, and Sutro had it rebuilt two years later. The Sutro Cliff House was the magnificent, cliff-hanging Victorian beauty so often featured in historic photos. Unfortunately, the most familiar of those photos is the 1907 shot of the building going up in flames. The current Cliff House, completed in 1909, is much less comely from the street but after a recent remodel has become a fine-looking restaurant and bistro, with exotic Casablanca décor and picture windows making the most of the sea view. If you're not eating, walk on through, find your way to the veranda overlooking the cliffs, and maybe plop some coins into the Camera Obscura for a large 360-degree view of the scenery. The big camera is mostly remarkable as a relic of archaic technology. The Camera Obscura represents a link in the chain of inventions that led to photography; Leonardo da Vinci drew up plans for such a device in the 15th century. Part of the scenery conveyed by the camera's lens includes Seal Rocks, where sea lions have long basked. Their numbers have dwindled in recent years, though, as the sea lions have migrated into the bay, where they laze about on the boat docks of Pier 39.

● Back out on the sidewalk, head north, to Louis' Restaurant. It's a casual and friendly diner with the same exceptional views you'd enjoy at the much more expensive Cliff House.

Back Story: Adolph Sutro

Adolf Sutro (1830–1898), a native of Prussia, moved to San Francisco during the Gold Rush and made his fortune on the Comstock Lode. He was an engineer, and his ticket to glory was in developing a tunnel that drained and ventilated the deep silver mines around Virginia City, Nevada. When Sutro sold his tunnel in 1879, he turned his attention to real estate in the rapidly growing city of San Francisco. He bought nearly 10 percent of the land within the city limits, most of it undeveloped at the time. Sutro served one term as the city's mayor, from 1894 to 1898. He termed himself the "anti-octopus" candidate, referring to the power of the Southern Pacific Railroad, which at the time was a many-tentacled political force.

- Just past Louis', a trail leads down to the Sutro Baths, one of San Francisco's more fascinating historic sites. Walk all the way down into the cove where long-abandoned swimming pools have become desolate duck ponds. You'll have to use your imagination (and refer to more old photos) to get an idea how awesome the Sutro Baths were when they opened in 1896. While walking (carefully) among the ruins, see if you can picture a massive steel framework supporting a glass dome overhead, with several large pools, slides, three restaurants, and a grandstand that seated 3,700. The water in each pool was a different temperature, and some pools contained salt water while others had fresh water. The baths were exceedingly popular for awhile, but by the late 1930s attendance had declined and the facility was converted into an ice rink. It closed in 1952 and burned down in 1966. (Lots of fires around these parts.) Make your way back up to the street. At the top of the steps turn left and walk through the parking lot to the Coastal Trail. We'll follow a small portion of the Coastal Trail, which runs for stretches up and down the state of California. Here, the trail hems fairly closely to the cliffs, overlooking the rocks and surf below. During low tide you can see the remains of three shipwrecks. If some parts of the trail pass through cleared land, it's due to a GGNRA program that is removing nonnative plants in order to encourage a return of native species.

- The trail skirts the western edge of Lincoln Park; a few hundred yards up, a spur leads right to the Palace of the Legion of Honor, one of the city's biggest art museums. Intriguingly, the building is a replica of a replica. The 1915 Panama Pacific Exposition included a French Pavilion, modeled on the Palais de la Légion d'Honneur in Paris. The French Pavilion showcased French art during the expo, then was torn down afterwards. Alma Spreckels, wife of sugar magnate Adolf Spreckels, missed the pavilion and had this more permanent version built. It opened in 1924. The museum's holdings include many 20th-century European masterpieces. You don't need to enter to have a look at Rodin's *The Thinker,* in front. It's a bronze cast, but Rodin oversaw its production. Some memorable scenes from Hitchcock's *Vertigo* were shot here.

- If it's nice beach weather, you can opt to hit a couple of beaches rather than visit the museum. To get to China Beach, take the Coastal Trail to McLaren Ave. and into the Richmond District. Follow it as it curves to the left and then hits Sea Cliff Ave. You'll see some steps leading down to the beach. China Beach, so named for the camp of

Chinese fishermen based here prior to the '06 quake, has swimmable surf, if you can stand the cold temperatures.

● Farther down Sea Cliff, where the street ends, a footpath (actually a continuation of the Coastal Trail) leads into the Presidio and to Baker Beach. This is the city's prime sunbathing spot, with a spectacular view of the sea, the Golden Gate, and the bridge. Swimming is not advisable, due to dangerous riptides. From here you can walk the sands almost all the way to the Golden Gate Bridge.

POINTS OF INTEREST

Cliff House **1090 Point Lobos Ave., 415-386-3330**

Louis' Restaurant **902 Point Lobos Ave., 415-387-6330**

Palace of the Legion of Honor **Lincoln Park, 34th Ave. and Clement St., 415-863-3330**

ROUTE SUMMARY

1. Start at Sutro Heights Park.
2. Walk down the path to Point Lobos Ave. and cross to the Cliff House.
3. From the Cliff House, go north, back up Point Lobos Ave., and head down the trail to the Sutro Baths.
4. From the Sutro Baths, return to the street and turn left, into the parking lot.
5. At the end of the parking lot, continue down the Coastal Trail.
6. A few hundred yards up the trail, turn right into Lincoln Park and the Palace of the Legion of Honor.
7. Return to the Coastal Trail and continue all the way until the trail meets McLaren Ave.
8. Follow McLaren Ave. as it curves left; where it meets Sea Cliff Ave., turn down the trail to China Beach.
9. From China Beach, take the trail back up to Sea Cliff Ave. and turn left.
10. At the end of Sea Cliff Ave. follow the trail down to Baker Beach.

Remnants of the Sutro Baths

Appendix 1: WalKS BY THeMe

architecture

Financial District (Walks 1 and 3)
Nob Hill (Walk 10)
Golden Gate Bridge (Walk 17)
Pacific Heights (Walk 18)
Market St. (Walks 1 and 26)

arts & culture

Union Square (Walk 4)
Civic Center (Walk 12)
Embarcadero South (Walk 19)
SOMA (Walk 20)
Mission Murals (Walk 22)

DINING, SHOPPING & entertainment

North Beach (Walks 7 and 8)
Tenderloin (Walk 13)
Mission Bars (Walk 23)
Castro (Walk 26)
Haight (Walk 29)
Japantown (Walk 31)
Richmond District (Walk 32)

HISTORY

Barbary Coast (Walk 6)
Market St. (Walks 1 and 26)

urBan ParKS

Marina (Walk 15)
Presidio (Walk 16 and 17)
Bernal Heights (Walk 24)
Glen Park (Walk 25)
Twin Peaks (Walk 27)
Corona Heights & Buena Vista Park
   (Walk 28)
Golden Gate Park (Walk 30)
Lands End (Walk 33)

stairways

Telegraph Hill (Walk 9)
Russian Hill (Walk 11)
Twin Peaks (Walk 27)

Appendix 2: POINTS OF INTEREST

FOOD & DRINK

Absinthe Brasserie and Bar 398 Hayes St., 415-551-1590 (Walk 12)

Balboa Cafe 3199 Fillmore St., 415-921-3944 (Walk 15)

Bambuddha Lounge 601 Eddy St., 415-885-5088 (Walk 13)

BaoNecci 516 Green St., 415-989-1806 (Walk 7)

Beach Chalet 1000 Great Highway, 415-386-8439 (Walk 30)

Bechelli's 2346 Chestnut St., 415-346-1801 (Walk 15)

Bix 56 Gold St, 415-433-6300 (Walk 6)

BlueJay Cafe 919 Divisadero St., 415-447-6066 (Walk 28)

Boudin Bakery 160 Jefferson St, 415-928-1849 (Walk 14)

Boulevard Restaurant Mission St, 415-543-6084 (Walk 19)

Bruno's 2389 Mission St., 415-643-5200 (Walk 23)

Buena Vista Cafe 2765 Hyde St, 415-474-5044 (Walk 14)

Burma Super Star 309 Clement St., 415-387-2147 (Walk 32)

Cafe Abir 1300 Fulton St., 415-567-7654 (Walk 28)

Café Bastille 22 Belden Place, 415-986-5673 (Walk 3)

Caffè Centro 102 South Park St., 415-882-1500

Cafe Flore 2298 Market St., 415-621-8579 (Walk 26)

Cafe Zoetrope 916 Kearny St., 415-291-1700 (Walk 7)

Caffè Trinity 1145 Market St., 415-626-2346 (Walk 1)

Caffe Macaroni 59 Columbus Ave., 415-956-9737 (Walk 7)

Caffè Trieste 601 Vallejo St, 415-392-6739 (Walk 7)

Capp's Corner 1600 Powell St., 415-989-2589 (Walk 7)

Chan Chan Café Cubano 4690 18th St., 415-864-4199 (Walk 27)

Cliff House 1090 Point Lobos Ave., 415-386-3330 (Walk 33)

FOOD & DRINK (CONTINUED)

Elite Cafe 2049 Fillmore St., 415-346-8668 (Walk 18)

Enrico's 504 Broadway, 415-982-6223 (Walk 7)

Farallon 450 Post St., 415-956-6969 (Walk 4)

Fisherman's Grotto No 9 9 Fisherman's Wharf, 415-673-7025 (Walk 14)

Fog City Diner 1300 Battery St., 415-982-2000 (Walk 2)

Foreign Cinema 534 Mission St., 415-648-7600 (Walk 23)

Gold Mountain 644 Broadway, 415-296-7733 (Walk 5)

Golden Era Vegetarian Restaurant 572 O'Farrell St., 415-673-3136 (Walk 13)

Golden Gate Bakery 1029 Grant Ave., 415-781-2627

Golden Gate Fortune Cookie Company 56 Ross Alley, 415-781-3956 (Walk 5)

Grand Cafe 501 Geary St., 415-292-0101 (Walk 4)

Greens Fort Mason Center, Building A, 415-771-6222 (Walk 15)

Jackson Fillmore 2506 Fillmore St., 415-346-5288 (Walk 18)

John's Grill 63 Ellis St., 415-986-3274

Kabuto Sushi 5121 Geary Blvd., 415-752-5652 (Walk 32)

Kan Zaman 1793 Haight St., 415-751-9656 (Walk 29)

La Palma Mexica-tessen 2884 24th St., 415-647-1500 (Walk 22)

La Taquería 2889 Mission St., 415-285-7117 (Walk 22)

Lefty O'Doul's 333 Geary St., 415-982-8900 (Walk 4)

Liberty Cafe 10 Cortland Ave., 415-695-8777 (Walk 24)

Liguria 1700 Stockton St., 415-421-3786 (Walk 7)

Lime 2247 Market St., 415-621-5256 (Walk 26)

Louis' Restaurant 902 Point Lobos Ave., 415-387-6330 (Walk 33)

Magnolia Pub & Brewery 1398 Haight St., 415-864-7468 (Walk 29)

Medjool 2522 Mission St., 415-550-9055 (Walk 23)

Minh's Garden 208 Clement St., 415-751-8211 (Walk 32)

Moki's Sushi and Pacific Grill 615 Cortland Ave., 415-970-9336 (Walk 24)

Molinari Delicatessen 373 Columbus Ave., 415-421-2337 (Walk 7)

Naked Lunch 504 Broadway, 415-577-4951 (Walk 8)

Old Ship Saloon 298 Pacific Ave., 415-788-2222 (Walk 2)

Pier 23 Cafe Pier 23, 415-362-5125 (Walk 2)

Pinecrest Diner 401 Geary St., 415-885-6407 (Walk 4)

Plouf 40 Belden Place, 415-986-6491 (Walk 3)

Red's Java House Pier 30, 415-777-5626 (Walk 19)

Rose Pistola 532 Columbus Ave., 415-399-0499 (Walk 7)

Sam's Grill 374 Bush St., 415-421-0594 (Walk 3)

Sam Wo Restaurant 813 Washington St., 415-982-0596 (Walk 5)

Sears' Fine Foods 439 Powell St., 415-986-0700 (Walk 4)

Slanted Door 1 Ferry Building, 415-861-8032 (Walk 2)

St. Francis Fountain 2801 24th St., 415-826-4200 (Walk 22)

South Park Cafe 108 South Park St., 415-495-7275

Tadich Grill 240 California St., 415-391-1849 (Walk 3)

Tad's Steaks 120 Powell St., 415-982-1718 (Walk 4)

Taquería Can-Cun 2288 Mission St., 415-252-9560 (Walk 22)

Tommy's Mexican Restaurant 5929 Geary Blvd., 415-387-4747 (Walk 22)

Ton Kiang 5821 Geary Blvd., 415-386-8530 (Walk 32)

Toy Boat Dessert Cafe 401 Clement St., 415-751-7505 (Walk 32)

Vietnam II 701 Larkin St., 415-885-1274 (Walk 13)

Warming Hut Crissy Field, 415-561-3040 (Walk 16)

Yank Sing 101 Spear St, 415-957-9300 (Walk 19)

HOTELS

Archbishop's Mansion 1000 Fulton St., 415-563-7872 (Walk 28)

Argonaut Hotel 495 Jefferson St., 415-563-0800 (Walk 14)

The Chateau Tivoli 1057 Steiner St., 415-776-5462 (Walk 28)

Fairmont Hotel 950 Mason St., 415-772-5000 (Walk 10)

Hotel Kabuki 1625 Post St., 415-922-3200 (Walk 31)

Hotel Triton 324 Grant Ave., 415-394-0500 (Walk 4)

Hyatt Regency 5 Embarcadero Center, 415-788-1234 (Walk 1)

HOTELS (CONTINUED)

Mark Hopkins Hotel 999 California St., 415-392-3434 (Walk 10)

Palace Hotel 2 New Montgomery St., 415-512-1111 (Walk 1)

Phoenix Hotel 601 Eddy St., 415-776-1380 (Walk 13)

Red Victorian B&B 1665 Haight St., 415-864-1978 (Walk 29)

Westin St. Francis Hotel 335 Powell St., 415-397-7000 (Walk 4)

ENTERTAINMENT & NIGHTLIFE

Atlas Cafe 3049 20th St., 415-648-1047 (Walk 23)

Aunt Charlie's Lounge 133 Turk St., 415-441-2922 (Walk 13)

Bimbo's 365 Club 1025 Columbus Ave., 415-474-0365 (Walk 11)

Boom Boom Room 1601 Fillmore St., 415-673-8000 (Walk 31)

Cafe Du Nord 2170 Market St., 415-861-5016 (Walk 26)

Castro Theater 429 Castro St., 415-621-6120 (Walk 26)

Comstock Saloon 155 Columbus Ave, 415-617-0071 (Walk 6)

Condor Club 560 Broadway, 415-781-8222 (Walk 6)

Doc's Clock 2575 Mission St., 415-824-3627 (Walk 23)

Edinburgh Castle 950 Geary St., 415-885-4074 (Walk 13)

Elbo Room 647 Valencia St., 415-552-7788 (Walk 23)

15 Romolo 15 Romolo Pl, 415-398-1359 (Walk 8)

Fillmore Auditorium 1805 Geary Blvd., 415-346-6000 (Walk 31)

Gangway 841 Larkin St., 415-776-6828 (Walk 13)

Gino and Carlo 548 Green St., 415-421-0896 (Walk 8)

Gold Dust Lounge 247 Powell St., 415-397-1695 (Walk 4)

Great American Music Hall 859 O'Farrell St., 415-885-0750 (Walk 13)

Ha Ra 875 Geary St., 415-673-3148 (Walk 13)

Hi Dive Pier 28-1/2, 415-977-0170 (Walk 19)

Latin American Club 3286 22nd St., 415-647-2732 (Walk 23)

Lusty Lady 1033 Kearny St., 415-391-3991 (Walk 6)

Make-Out Room 3225 22nd St., 415-647-2888 (Walk 23)

Mario's Bohemian Cigar Store 566 Columbus Ave., 415-362-0536 (Walk 8)

Mint Karaoke Lounge 1942 Market St., 415-626-4726 (Walk 26)

Mitchell Bros. O'Farrell Theater 895 O'Farrell St., 415-776-6686 (Walk 13)

Perry's 1944 Union St., 415-922-9022 (Walk 15)

Pied Piper Bar 2 New Montgomery St., 415-512-1111 (Walk 1)

The Plough and the Stars 116 Clement St., 415-751-1122 (Walk 32)

Purple Onion 140 Columbus Ave., 415-956-1610 (Walk 7)

Rite Spot Cafe 2099 Folsom St., 415-552-6066 (Walk 23)

Saloon 1232 Grant Ave., 415-989-7666 (Walk 8)

Specs' 12 William Saroyan Place, 415-421-4112 (Walk 8)

Starlight Room 450 Powell St., 415-395-8595 (Walk 4)

Tonga Room 950 Mason St., 415-772-5278 (Walk 10)

Tony Nik's 1534 Stockton St., 415-693-0993 (Walk 8)

Top of the Mark 999 California St., 415-616-6916 (Walk 10)

Tosca Cafe 242 Columbus Ave., 415-391-1244 (Walk 8)

Trad'r Sam 6150 Geary Blvd., 415-221-0773 (Walk 32)

Tunnel Top 601 Bush St., 415-986-8900 (Walk 4)

Twin Peaks Tavern 401 Castro St., 415-864-9470 (Walk 26)

Uptown 200 Capp St., 415-861-8231 (Walk 23)

Vesuvio 255 Columbus Ave., 415-362-3370 (Walk 8)

Wild Side West 424 Cortland Ave., 415-647-3099 (Walk 24)

Zeitgeist 199 Valencia St., 415-255-7505 (Walk 23)

MUSEUMS & GALLERIES

Asian Art Museum 200 Larkin St., 415-581-3500 (Walk 12)

Beat Museum 540 Broadway, 800-537-6822 (Walk 7)

Cable Car Museum 1201 Mason St., 415-474-1887 (Walk 10)

California Academy of Sciences 55 Music Concourse Dr., 415-379-8000

California Historical Society 678 Mission St., 415-357-1848 (Walk 20)

MUSEUMS & GALLERIES (CONTINUED)

Cartoon Art Museum 655 Mission St., 415-227-8666 (Walk 20)

The Chinese Historical Society of America 965 Clay St., 415-391-1188 (Walk 5)

Galería de la Raza 2857 24th St., 415-826-8009 (Walk 22)

M.H. De Young Memorial Museum 50 Hagiwara Tea Garden Dr., 415-863-3330 (Walk 30)

Musée Mécanique Pier 45 Shed A, 415-346-2000

Museum of the African Diaspora (MoAD) 685 Mission St., 415-358-7200 (Walk 20)

Palace of the Legion of Honor Lincoln Park, 34th Ave. and Clement St., 415-863-3330 (Walk 33)

San Francisco Arts Commission Gallery 401 Van Ness Ave., 415-554-6080 (Walk 12)

San Francisco Museum of Modern Art (SFMoMA) 151 Third St., 415-357-4000 (Walk 20)

San Francisco National Maritime Museum 900 Beach St., 415-561-7100 (Walk 14)

Walt Disney Family Museum 104 Montgomery St., 415-345-6800 (Walk 16)

Wells Fargo History Museum 420 Montgomery St., 415-396-2619 (Walk 3)

Yerba Buena Center for the Arts 701 Mission St., 415-978-2787 (Walk 20)

EDUCATIONAL & CULTURAL CENTERS

The Center 1800 Market St., 415-865-5555 (Walk 26)

Exploratorium 3601 Lyon St., 415-563-7337 (Walk 15)

Hyde St. Pier 415-447-5000 (Walk 14)

Main Library 100 Larkin St., 415-557-4400 (Walk 12)

Maritime Visitor Center Hyde and Jefferson Sts., 415-447-5000 (Walk 14)

Precita Eyes Art Store & Visitors Center 2981 24th St., 415-285-2287 (Walk 22)

San Francisco Art Institute 800 Chestnut St., 415-771-7020 (Walk 11)

HISTORICAL LANDMARKS & MONUMENTS

Bank of Canton (Old Chinese Telephone Exchange) 743 Washington St. (Walk 5)

City Club 155 Sansome St., 415-648-7198 (Walk 3)

Coit Tower 1 Telegraph Hill Blvd., 415-362-0808 (Walk 9)

Colonial Dames Octagon House 2645 Gough St., 415-441-7512 (Walk 15)

Haas-Lilienthal House 2007 Franklin St., 415-441-3004 (Walk 18)

Masonic Memorial Temple 1111 California St., 415-776-4702 (Walk 10)

Officers' Club (NPS Visitors Center) Presidio, 415-561-4323 (Walk 16)

Redstone Building 2926 16th St. (Walk 22)

San Francisco Columbarium 1 Loraine Court (Walk 32)

SS *Jeremiah O'Brien* Pier 45, 415-544-0100 (Walk 14)

USS *Pampanito* Pier 45, 415-561-7006 (Walk 14)

Women's Building 3543 18th St., 415-431-1180 (Walk 22)

PLaCes OF WORSHIP

Buddhist Church 1881 Pine St. (Walk 31)

Grace Cathedral 1100 California St., 415-749-6300 (Walk 10)

Konko Kyo Church 1909 Bush St., 415-931-0453 (Walk 31)

Mission Dolores 3321 16th St., 415-621-8203 (Walk 21)

Notre Dame des Victoires 566 Bush St., 415-397-0113 (Walk 4)

Sts. Peter and Paul Church 666 Filbert St., 415-421-0809 (Walk 7)

Vedanta Temple 2963 Webster St., 415-922-2323 (Walk 15)

SHOPPING

A Different Light Bookstore 489 Castro St., 415-431-0891 (Walk 26)

Aria 1522 Grant Ave., 415-433-0219 (Walk 7)

Book Bay Fort Mason, Fort Mason Center, Building C, 415-771-1076 (Walk 15)

Bound Together Book Collective 1369 Haight St., 415-431-8355 (Walk 29)

Canton Bazaar 616 Grant Ave., 415-362-5750 (Walk 5)

Casa Lucas Market 2934 24th St., 415-593-0785 (Walk 22)

SHOPPING (CONTINUED)

City Lights Books 261 Columbus Ave., 415-362-8193 (Walk 7)

Clarion Music Center 816 Sacramento St., 415-391-1317 (Walk 5)

Cliff's Variety Store 479 Castro St., 415-431-5365 (Walk 26)

Green Apple Books and Music 506 Clement St., 415-387-2272 (Walk 32)

Kamei Housewares and Restaurant Supplies 525–547 Clement St., 415-666-3688 (Walk 32)

Kayo Books 814 Post St., 415-749-0554 (Walk 13)

Kinokuniya Bookstore 1581 Webster St., 415-567-7625 (Walk 31)

Mario's Bohemian Cigar Store 566 Columbus Ave., 415-362-0536

Marcus Books 1712 Fillmore St., 415-346-4222 (Walk 31)

Mission Market Fish & Poultry 2590 Mission St., 415-282-3331 (Walk 22)

New May Wah Supermarket 719 Clement St., 415-221-9826 (Walk 32)

Nijiya Market 1737 Post St., 415-563-1901 (Walk 31)

Pipe Dreams 1376 Haight St., 415-431-3553 (Walk 29)

Positively Haight Street 1400 Haight St., 415-252-8747 (Walk 29)

Red Blossom Tea Company 831 Grant Ave., 415-395-0868 (Walk 5)

Soul Patch Tattoo and Piercing 1599 Haight St., 415-552-3444 (Walk 29)

Wasteland 1660 Haight St., 415-863-3150 (Walk 29)

PARKS & GARDENS

Conservatory of Flowers John F. Kennedy Dr., 415-666-7001 (Walk 30)

Hagiwara Japanese Tea Garden Hagiwara Tea Garden Dr., 415-831-2700 (Walk 30)

Strybing Arboretum & Botanical Gardens 9th Ave. at Lincoln Way, 415-661-1316 (Walk 30)

MISCELLANEOUS

AT&T Park 24 Willie Mays Plaza (corner Third and King), 415-972-1800 (Walk 19)

INDEX

aBOUT THE auTHOr

Tom Downs grew up in the Santa Clara Valley, south of San Francisco. He has lived in Los Angeles, New York City, Oakland, and Berkeley, as well as in Chinatown and the Mission District in San Francisco. He is a travel writer who has authored books and articles about New Orleans, Hanoi, and the West of Ireland for Lonely Planet, the BBC Worldwide, and a host of magazines, newspapers, and websites. His photography has appeared in countless publications, including *National Geographic* and *The New York Times*. In 2007 his post-Katrina New Orleans was honored with the Lowell Thomas Award, granted by the Society of American Travel Writers, for Best Guidebook. Tom says he wore out dozens of pairs of shoes compiling the material for this book, and he expects to go through many more pairs in the years ahead.